PSYCHING UP

Also by Julius Fast

The Beatles: The Real Story
Body Language
The Pleasure Book
The Body Language of Sex, Power, and Aggression

PSYCHING UP

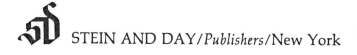

OVER 50
GOOD IDEAS
FOR A
SLIMMER,
SEXIER,
HEALTHIER
YOU

Julius Fast

sD STEIN AND DAY/*Publishers*/New York

First published in 1978
Copyright © 1978 by Julius Fast
All rights reserved
Designed by Karen Bernath
Printed in the United States of America
Stein and Day/*Publishers*/Scarborough House,
Briarcliff Manor, N.Y. 10510

Library of Congress Cataloging in Publication Data

Fast, Julius, 1919–
   Psyching up

    1. Hygiene.   2. Diet.   3. Sex.   4. Pleasure.
I. Title.
RA776.5.F37   613   76-46584
ISBN 0-8128-2154-8

For Jack and Moira

Contents

Introduction

"I am a little like the man who found it easy to give up cigarettes," Vern told me. "He found it so easy that he did it time and again. I find it very easy to diet—I do it so often."

When I pressed my friend, he admitted that while he started each diet with enthusiasm, he never stuck with it. "I lose a few pounds and then it's all downhill. It gets so boring. I'm seduced from grace by an ice cream cone or a chocolate eclair. What I need is a diet with excitement."

"I have some friends," I told him, "who lost weight with ice cream sundaes and gourmet food, and stuck with their diet."

Vern lifted his eyebrows. "Now, that I've got to hear. Do you think it would help me?"

"I think it would. What you need, it seems to me, is some way of psyching yourself up to a proper diet." I explained the basics of the Saturday Sundae diet to him, and he nodded happily. "You know, I could go with that—in fact, it might be a lot of fun."

In the weeks that passed, Vern did go with it, and to his amazement took off all the weight he had wanted to lose. "Now, to keep it off," he told me, "but that's another story."

I wondered if it was. Vern's diet—the Saturday Sundae diet—was basically an ordinary low-calorie diet, but psyched up by the gourmet foods it included. It was a diet for someone who needed sensations. Vern was like that. In fact, he was what Professor Marvin Zukerman of the University of Delaware has characterized as a "High Sensation Seeker." In a study of why people search for sensations, Dr. Zukerman found that many of us have an innate need for more stimulation than others. They aren't driven by compulsive neurotic needs, he assures us. They simply have a very strong response to new stimuli, and probably a low level of toleration for the ordinary. Like Vern, they become bored with the humdrum quality of daily life. They look for something different, something more exciting, more stimulating, a way of psyching up their reactions.

The strange thing is that all too often what they consider the extraordinary consists of nothing more than the very ordinary looked at from a different angle. Turning the corner of perception can give anyone a startling view of a familiar landscape.

For many people, sex can become routine and dull—and yet a minimal change, a different place, a touch of fantasy, a bit of dress-up, can turn routine sex into thrilling sex.

The same is true of exercise. Gyms and health clubs can be deadly bores, dull repetitions of the same movements, the same workouts day after day. But take your exercise out of the gym and into the home or outdoors. Add that different perception to it, and the dullness disappears. You're left with a sensational high.

While many of us are high sensation seekers, even those of us who aren't still need a great deal of psyching up in our ordinary life. I began to question my friends, and I was amazed to find out how many people had secret techniques for psyching themselves up to diet or exercise—or even sex. A few had ways of getting high without drugs or alcohol, new techniques of massage or tricks of chanting, pampering themselves with baths and facials, or, as one trim young man explained, "A secret exercise I'll never let anyone watch!"

In every case, I found that there was nothing very extraordinary about these personal highs. The only extraordinary thing was the altered state of consciousness each high brought, the psyching-up process that allowed people to take a dull routine and turn it into something intriguing and unusual.

The main point of this book is to share with you all the secrets of the people I interviewed. I talked to hundreds and then selected the most unusual, but still those whose tricks and techniques were available to all of us. I hope that once you share these experiences by reading, you'll try some. I know I have, and it's been a time of discovery and pleasure—and in many cases a shortcut to health.

This is a book for browsing. You can open it at random and share the different sensations of the people who shared their secrets with me. Think about each and try those you dare. If you are afraid to try them—and many of you will be out of shyness, fear, or preference—then at least fantasize a bit and try to share the forbidden highs in daydreams. You may very well find enough secret enjoyment that way to try a few of them in real life.

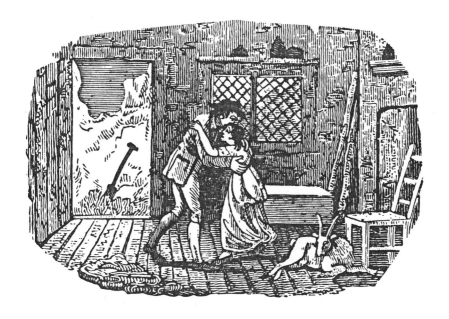

LOVE IN THE AFTERNOON

The pressures of a hectic job, young children, and other commitments had taken some of the fun out of sex for one couple. Here's how they used a logistical change to make sex sexier.

"When I was a teen-ager," Richie tells me, "I'd think nothing of traveling fifty, even a hundred miles to make out with a girl. I remember once driving all the way up to Boston from New York just to spend a couple of hours with some very cute chick."

"Was it worth it?"

"Of course. We had great sex going, the two of us—though for the life of me I can't remember her name now. But you know, I still remember the anticipation on the drive up there and the memory of it on the way back. One thing for sure—it was worth it.

Richie says seriously, "That's why now that I'm married, I think nothing of taking the subway home during my lunch break to get together with my wife."

"But it's a half-hour each way!"

Grinning, Richie says, "My wife picks me up at the station. The kids are off at school, and we have a matinee."

"A matinee?"

"Sex in the afternoon! There's nothing like it. Look, the usual routine is sex at night, but at night Margie and I are both too tired. She's had the kids all afternoon—cooking and cleaning—it's rough, I know, and I've had the office, fighting the rush hour to get home, still angry over some client or other—and then there are all the little jobs around the house.... By bedtime we're both exhausted, and if we want sex, which we rarely do by then, we have to force ourselves. And then there are the kids. We have to wait till they get to sleep, and by then we're both pooped even if we were feeling good before."

"What about the mornings?"

"Hah!" He snorts. "They're no better. Margie doesn't really come alive till after ten, and I'm racing to get to work and get the kids off to school—the mornings are mad. If we do wake up early—and it's rare for both of us to do that—we're nervous about the kids barging in, about getting breakfast ready—no, we're both too much on edge in the morning to enjoy ourselves.

"But by twelve o'clock things have fallen into place. Marge has the house in order. She's relaxed and has taken care of all the bothersome jobs around the house. The kids are off at school, and I've finished a good morning's work. I tell my secretary I'm taking a long lunch break—important client, I hint with a vague shrug—and I hurry over to the subway.

"It's never crowded at that hour, and I can relax, read my newspaper or a book, and get myself into the same anticipatory frame of mind I used to have when I was a kid driving up to Boston. Marge meets me at the station, and we're home in a few minutes.

"We dial our own number on the telephone so it'll be busy to anyone trying to reach Marge. We lock the door and we hurry upstairs."

"But so much effort for—for just marital sex," I protest. "It seems way overdone."

"Ah!" Richie smiles. "That's just it. You see, with that much effort, it's not just marital sex. It becomes something special, something different and unusual. We don't have our matinees too often. They never become routine, and the very fact that it's an effort sets it apart.

"And besides, there's something vaguely illicit about it all. It's as if we were cheating everyone by sneaking in this little matinee. It becomes a special secret—our secret.

"It's a bit like it was when we first met and we had to go through all kinds of obstacles—fooling Margie's mother and my folks, too, just to get into bed with each other. That, for all the hassle, was fun, and we recapture that fun. Then, sometimes I bring flowers home at noon, and once I picked up a bottle of champagne. We iced it in the freezer and afterward had a toast to illicit love before I went back to work.

"You see, the entire mood of sex during a matinee is different, freer, and yet a little wicked—as if we were lovers instead of man and wife. Hell, I know any number of guys who would think nothing of sneaking off to a hotel with another woman during a lunch break . . . as long as it wasn't their wife. So I sneak off to my wife."

He snapped his fingers. "Hey, speaking of hotels, last summer when the kids were home, I took a room at a hotel near the office and Marge got a sitter for the kids and drove into town. We figured that that was doing it with class. You know, we were both sure everyone in the hotel suspected we were lovers instead of husband and wife—at least it seemed that way to us."

Nodding, I say, "You know, I see how it could be fun. I think I'll try it."

"Go ahead. You'll like it." Richie shook his head. "I guarantee it'll spark up a tired marriage—and make a good one better, or at least more fun."

What if you and your spouse both work? That's even better! As long as you both work in the same general area, it's even easier to arrange a matinee get-together at a hotel. Take advantage of the special hourly rates offered by many reputable hotels and motels. You may feel a bit sheepish checking in, but you'll feel great checking out.

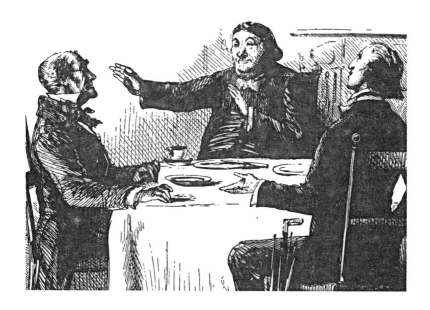

THE DIETING
GAME

Dieting can be fun—if you make it into a game. Play by the rules and you'll always win.

I saw Derek at dinner at a friend's house six months after his heart attack, and it took a long, hard look before I could recognize him. "My God, you've changed!"

"For better or worse?"

"For the better, of course. You look ten years younger."

He stroked his handsome gray moustache and smiled. "I think it gives me a touch of *je ne sais quoi.*"

"Not your moustache. It's your weight. You're half of what you used to be."

Only a few inches over five feet tall, Derek used to have an untidy body. He always walked with a spring, for all his weight, and he gave the illusion of bouncing into a room. Now he was a different Derek, altogether slim and trim and very elegant.

After dinner, I cornered him in our hostess's den. "Was it very difficult, taking the weight off?" I asked.

"Difficult? Not really, at least not any more, not in keeping it off. There's so much enjoyment I get out of my diet."

"That's a new one!"

"Well, you've got to understand. Before I had my coronary, I lived a pretty hectic life. I headed our PR firm, and the stress was something you wouldn't believe. I handled it by eating and drinking. For me, food was a pacifier. You know how much I weighed the night I had my heart attack? Twice what I weigh now. *Twice!*"

I remembered Derek in the hospital, bare-chested and half-sitting up in bed, with tubes and wires plugged into a monitoring device, for all the world like a giant computerized Buddha.

"I think I began to enjoy food in the hospital after I got out of intensive care, once they put me on a very bland diet."

"How do you mean, enjoy? Didn't you enjoy food before?"

"I enjoyed eating, but food?" He bit his lip. "Did I really enjoy it? I felt compelled to eat. I think that's it. Food was like an addiction, but I didn't care what I ate. I don't believe I ever really tasted it." He shook his head. "I always ate well, expensive restaurants—you know the expense account I had— and Carol is one hell of a cook. The night I had the attack, I had demolished one of her roasts—the kind she makes with pastry crust and liver."

"Beef Wellington?"

"Could be. I was so busy eating it, I never had time to name it. Well, the point is, I never really appreciated the fine taste of food, the subtle tastes. I flooded my gut with spices and sauces and elaborate dishes. I drowned my taste.

"In the hospital, after they knew I was going to make it, they put me on a strict salt-free diet of 1,000 calories a day with only 60 grams of carbohydrates, and they told me I'd have to stay on it for at least a year. I tell you, I was kind of stunned at that. Also the bland diet I was getting then. I couldn't imagine how I'd cope with it.

"But the crazy thing is. I really enjoyed it. You see, I've known I was overweight for how long? Twenty years? My doctor was always after me to diet—Carol, too—but she couldn't stop cooking the stuff she does, and I just didn't have the drive or willpower to stop eating." He shrugged. "Or motivation, I guess."

"A heart attack is pretty strong motivation."

"Especially when you have no choice in the matter, like in the hospital. That's where I got my start. They furnished the discipline and the menu."

"I know those hospital menus!"

"Well, that's the funny part. With a really bland diet, I began to enjoy things I never enjoyed before. Like Jell-O. They served me the dietetic kind. After I got out of intensive care, they let me eat all I wanted, but they played a little game with me. My nurse pretended that I'd have trouble getting all I wanted, and she said she'd have to prescribe it as if it were a medicine. Later I found out that was nonsense, but I enjoyed playing the game. It was the first diet game I played, and I got to the point where I anticipated Jell-O as if it were a real treat—which it was.

"Cold cereal, too. I never used to eat cold cereal. My old breakfast used to be bacon or sausage and eggs, buttered muffins, maybe a stack of wheatcakes, coffee with cream and sugar—if I was at a hotel, I'd have fruit with cream on it.

"In the hospital I had my choice of cold cereal, and it was a new taste—and a boiled egg. Who ever ate a boiled egg in preference to a fried one? I used to order three-minute, four-minute and five-minute eggs until I realized that they were bringing me the same egg no matter what I ordered. I began to drink black coffee, too, and I realized that without that gummy cream and sugar coffee has a totally different taste—a good taste.

"Now I play games. I know I'm limited in what I can eat, but I juggle calories. I increase the amount I eat until there's the slightest weight gain. Then I cut back. Or I'll allow myself just enough food during the day so I don't get hungry—too hungry—and I'll splurge at dinner. Tonight I knew we'd have corn and I love corn, so I saved up my calories during the day."

"How often do you weigh yourself?" I asked.

"Oh, twice a day. My upper limit is 130 pounds. They thought it would take me a year to get down to that, but I made it in six months. Now I never let my weight get over that."

"Wouldn't you be better weighing yourself once a day?"

"Probably, but the twice-a-day routine is part of my anxiety. Eventually I'm sure I'll get over that. Another game I play is to get the most food I can out of my calories and carbohydrates."

"How do you do that?"

"I have a lot of time on my hands now—I'm still not back to a full workload—so I draw up menus."

"You mean menus that give you the most food?"

"Right. Like a typical breakfast menu might be two boiled eggs—that's 160 calories and no carbohydrates, three cups of coffee—no calories or carbohydrates, and a tablespoon of peanut butter—92 calories, but only two grams of carbohydrates."

"Peanut butter?"

"You think that's only for kids? I love peanut butter because it's so filling. One tablespoon fills me up as much as four slices of cheese."

"I don't know if I could take it. I haven't tasted peanut butter since—God knows when."

"Try it, you'll like it—but not the creamy kind. Try the chunky style. Now for lunch I might have some sardines in tomato sauce, about one and one-half sardines—that's 120 calories and no carbohydrates. I fill my plate with salad, 15 and 2. A tablespoon of imitation mayonnaise is 50 and one, or the dietetic salad dressing is 6 and one—that's calories and carbohydrates."

"I get it."

"For dinner I'll have four to six ounces of lean meat—that's 300 calories and zero on carbohydrates. I trim off all the fat. I have a small potato—75 and 10, a slice of bread—100 and 15, a green vegetable—20 and 5, and my old favorite dessert—Jell-O, 40 and zero.

"Then I balance it all up to see where I am in terms of my 1,000 calories and 60 grams of carbohydrates. I find I can afford a snack at bedtime. I've had only 972 calories and 34 grams of carbohydrates. A piece of fruit will run 50 and 10, cheese, 50 and 2—darned close to my 1,000 and 60 limits—and that's a diet guaranteed to take weight off anyone."

Derek shakes his head. "I know it's an involved diet, and maybe that's bad—but maybe it's good, too. I needed the involvement those months after my attack."

"What other games do you play?"

"Oh—the construction game. If the meal Carol prepares isn't in my calorie counter, I construct its value."

"How do you mean?"

"Well, for instance, none of the diet books tell you what's in shrimp parmigiana. I use analogies to find out. One book will tell you what veal parmigiana is, and then you find out the difference between shrimp and veal and subtract—I take this diet routine very seriously, I guess because of what happened to me. I weigh all my food—oh, not when we eat out, but by now I can approximate weight. The other day we ate out and I ordered a hamburger. I figured it would be about three, four ounces tops. It came and it was sixteen full ounces, a whole pound of meat! The restaurant was very proud of itself."

"And you?"

"I was disgusted with them and the kind of culture that pushes all that overconsumption. But I'd never have felt that way before. I ate my four ounces and left the rest—and I had to discipline myself to do it. I hated to leave all that food, but Carol finally came to my rescue and ordered a doggie bag to take it home."

"I guess your stomach has shrunk."

"No. That's the point. It's my mind, not my stomach. I'm very seldom full now, and if I had let myself go, I could have eaten all that meat. I ate a full dinner tonight, but I could easily sit down now and have a sandwich. I guess that's what makes a fat man. I'll always be one, no matter how thin I am."

While I was thinking about that, Derek said, "I'd do it again, you know."

Startled, I asked, "Do what? Have another heart attack?"

"Hell, no! I mean diet like that. Whatever caused me to do it, I feel freer now, more alive and aware—and I'm able to taste again, really taste all kinds of food, not just the overspiced, oversauced gourmet food I used to wallow in."

There was a knock at the door and our hostess called out, "You two. How about a brandy?"

"There." Derek stood up with a wry grin. "What's an average brandy? My mind ticks it out. Two ounces? 180 and 12—there's no way I'll stoke up on that. Me for a diet cola with a lot of ice!"

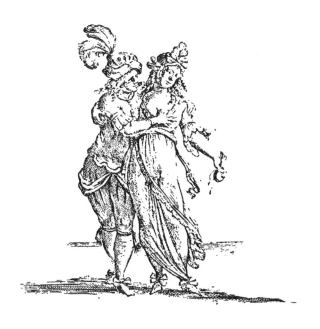

THE LOVE AFFAIR
OF YOUR DREAMS

If sexual fantasies can be fun, living out those dreams can be even more fun. Here's one way to add zest to any marriage.

I was coming home to my city apartment the other night, when I noticed a young woman, attractive, in her mid-twenties, with long blond hair, in a furious argument with a man about the same age. They were across the street from me, and as I came up to them, the argument exploded into action. The man pushed the girl roughly against a parked car, turned her to face the car and made her lean forward, her hands and feet spread-eagled.

I've seen Kojak, Starsky, and Hutch do that routine often enough on TV and I checked my impulse to cross over and interfere. Was this a genuine arrest? The young girl looked so innocent and vulnerable and frightened.

The man frisked her quickly, then pulled her away from the car and flashed his wallet, which must have contained a badge. I couldn't see it from where I stood. Then he bent her arm behind her and marched her toward the avenue.

I was so surprised at the entire routine that I stood there watching them until they came abreast of the house at the corner. Then the detecti e(?) released the woman's arm, slipped his own arm around her shoulder, kissed her, and guided her into the building!

What had I witnessed? I wondered in bewilderment as I turned and continued home. The answer came the next day. I was passing the corner house just as the same young man came out of it. I couldn't control my curiosity. I stopped him and asked, "Do you live here?"

Surprised, he looked at me and nodded. "Yes, I do. Why?"

"And the young lady you marched in here last night," I asked. "Does she live here, too? Forgive my curiosity, but what was that all about?"

To my surprise, he blushed a deep red and smiled uncomfortably. "It was really just a game," he said softly. "We—well, we live together, and it—" He shrugged uncomfortably. "It turns us both on."

I said, "Of course. I didn't mean to be nosy. It was just that watching it—well, it seemed to be so real."

He laughed at that, a bit more relaxed. "To us it was real."

I kept thinking about it for the rest of the day, the little charade that turned them both on. "Do you think," I asked a psychiatrist friend over coffee a few days later, "that such pretense, such game playing can actually—work?"

"Work how?" he asked. "In what way?"

"It seems to me that both of them must have gotten some sort of erotic charge out of the act."

"Of course, and why not?"

"You sound as if it's common. Don't they realize that it's only playacting? How can that excite them?"

"They realize it's all pretend, but that needn't take away

from the excitement of the act. I have a patient who's heavily into S and M, you know, sadism and masochism. He's the gentlest man you can imagine in real life, a regular Casper Milquetoast, but he and his wife play this sex game where he dresses up in a leather jacket, jeans, and motorcycle boots, and he knocks her about the bedroom, then drags her to the bed and rapes her."

"Rapes her?"

"While she begs him not to. It's an incredible turn-on for both of them. He says she has an orgasm the moment he enters her, and he gets so high he can barely contain himself. Of course they both know they're acting, and they both know he would never really hurt her, but they play out their favorite fantasy—and they play it out safely. That's the main point of these sexual charades—playing out your favorite fantasy safely."

The idea was intriguing, and after I left him, I began to wonder how many of my friends played this game. "More than you suspect," my wife told me. "Just the other day Gilda told me how she and her husband get their kicks."

"Tell me!" Gilda is in her forties, a very proper, rather rigid woman. The idea of Gilda getting "kicks" in any way seems strange.

"By fighting in public. She and her husband start an argument in the street, in a market, or even in a restaurant, and escalate it into a real shouting match all the way home. They get home pretending to be so furious with each other that they can hardly talk, and wham—sex! Gilda says it's absolutely wild. Pretending to fight like that excites both of them."

I shudder. "It would destroy me. I'd die of embarrassment if I ever had a public argument with you. And I'd be furious with you for allowing it. How the hell can that be sexually stimulating?"

"Each to his own. It works for Gilda and her husband." But Gilda, I find out later, is no exception. The games people play to turn on sexually are as varied as they are intriguing.

"We play out scenes from a book," a friend confided. "My

wife and I look for interludes, incidents, meetings, unusual scenes in literature that we can—well, I guess you'd call it dramatize. We act them out very seriously, and they work for us. It's like—like getting out of your own skin and into someone else's. You see, you can be anything if you're acting, and your partner can be anything or anyone that you find sexually exciting and provocative. Anyone—everything in life is a charade, isn't it?"

That's too good a statement to let go by, so we get into a long discussion about illusion and reality. Later, when I tell my wife about it, she looks at me thoughtfully. "You know what's happening, don't you?"

"No, tell me."

"You're so intrigued that you want to try the game, but you haven't the guts to admit it."

"Well, I'm not about to fight in public or pretend to frisk you on the street or rape you in the bedroom . . ."

"I'd get the giggles if you did—but I do have an idea."

"What is it?"

"There's a singles bar down the block. Let's both go."

"Together? To a singles bar?"

"No, silly, apart. We'll pretend to be single."

"Oh, great! At my age no one would pay any attention to me, and I'd be destroyed."

"But that's just it. There's one man who'd pick me up."

"Who's that?"

"You, stupid! Shall we try it?"

"Why not? Who goes first? Wait—I'd better. I'm not so sure that if you go in alone someone won't try to pick you up."

"Flattery will work every time. You go on while I get dressed."

The bar was very dark and very, very crowded. I felt a bit like Father Time. There wasn't anyone there over thirty! I pushed my way through and catching the bartender's eye ordered a beer. When it came, I clutched it for security and looked around. The eyes met mine and flicked away with all the disinterest I had suspected. But wait! Who had just come in the door?

I caught her eye across the dim room and held it. She had a disdainful look, but wasn't there a touch of uncertainty under that lovely, cool exterior? A touch of confusion?

I walked toward her carefully and said, "Let me buy you a drink."

Her eyes widened and she looked at me, aloof at first and then speculatively. "If you want to." Her voice was like ice in the hot, crowded bar.

I had a live one here! I shoved my way back to the bar wondering how long before I could say, very casually, "Your place or mine?"

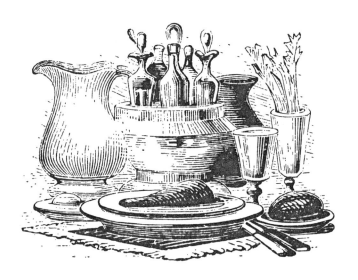

SATURDAY SUNDAE

Must dieting be unpleasant? Not at all, according to two former fatties who called their diet "a pleasure."

I run into Judy and John outside the local movie house, and after chatting about the picture, I suddenly realize that something has changed. As long as I've known them, this couple have been typical roly-polies, neither taller than 5'3" and both at least 50 pounds overweight. In our crowd they've been nicknamed Tweedledum and Tweedledee, and to see them waddle down the street together, hand in hand, you appreciate the nicknames at once.

Now, talking to them, I see that the old nickname no longer

fits. They are both almost normal in size. "What happened?" I ask. "Where did it all go?"

"Off, for good!" Judy says firmly. "We have dieted it all away, and we're going right down to bedrock."

"How far down is bedrock?"

"Another ten pounds."

Always intrigued by someone else's successful diet, I ask, "How did you do it? What diet did you use? Was it Weight Watchers, or Fatties Anonymous?"

I catch a sly look between the two. John shakes his head, and Judy evasively says, "It's much too complicated to explain here on a street corner. We'll get together one of these days and tell you all about it. We've got to run now."

Intrigued, I ask, "But was it very hard?"

John smiles briefly and mysteriously as they turn away. "Not at all. I found it all a pleasure."

I brood on the mystery for over a week, and then, stopping into the local ice cream shop one night, I find Judy and John in a corner booth bent over two enormous ice cream sundaes, expressions of absolute rapture on their faces.

I slide into the booth next to Judy and say, "So it's all off."

Startled, and with a guilty look, John looks up. "What's off?"

"Your diet. Your so-successful diet. A pleasure, I think you called it."

"Off? Of course it's not off!" he protests indignantly, but with a touch of embarrassment. "Judy and I are still dieting." He takes a spoonful of ice cream topped with chocolate sauce and whipped cream and eats it slowly, savoring it blissfully. I watch as he finishes and licks the spoon.

Judy stands up and smooths down her skirt around a pair of slim, shapely hips. "We're down three more pounds!" She sits again and picks up her spoon. "Does that look as if we're off the diet?"

"But I don't understand," I protest with a frown. "Here I catch you both out cheating on your diet—and what a cheat! Ice cream, chocolate sauce, whipped cream, even a cherry—and you say you're still dieting!"

"The whipped cream is from a spray can," John says smugly. "That means fewer calories. A lot of air, you know."

"The sundae is 589 calories, to be exact," Judy explains. "At least that's how I figure it."

"I round it out to 600," John nods.

"What's the difference between 589 and 600?" I say. "You're obviously breaking your diet, and I'll bet this isn't an isolated episode."

"You sound like Mrs. Beauregarde, my sixth-grade teacher, when she caught me smoking in the boy's room," John laughs. "An isolated episode indeed! How uptight can you get. Look, we're two adults. Do you think we'd cheat on a diet?"

"From where I sit, it looks as if you are. You'd better explain."

"Why don't you order for yourself? Here's the waitress," John suggests. "Then let's just concentrate on the sundaes before they melt."

I order a double dish of plain vanilla—I hate all that sauce they spoil ice cream with—and when it comes, Judy nods. "You could diet easily. You really don't like the high-calorie trim. But you could have had three scoops of ice cream."

I take her advice and don't talk until our plates are cleaned. Then I lean back and say, "All right, now give. Do you come here often?"

"Three or four nights a week, sometimes five, since we started dieting," John says, enjoying my confusion. "Before that we came here very rarely—only when we fell from grace— and then we would feel pretty guilty and furtive about it."

"You looked pretty guilty and furtive tonight."

"Old habits die slowly." John shrugged. "Even though it's legit, we still feel a bit uneasy."

"But how is it legit? Will you both stop teasing and tell me about this diet that lets you eat all the sundaes you want."

"We call it the gourmet delight diet," John said, "and it's really very simple. You know I'm in my thirties and pretty active. Now the government-recommended allowance of calories for someone in my age group who's as active as I am is over 3,000 a day."

"Government recommended? That sounds very official."

"The Food and Nutrition Board of the National Research Council. But any diet book will tell you the same thing. I simply cut down to 2,500 calories a day, and the weight comes off. That's it."

"That's it?" I look at the empty sundae dish and lift my eyebrows. "How does that fit in?"

"It figures to about 600 calories. The ice cream—half a pint— is 300. The chocolate sauce another 100. The whipped cream, if it were real would be about 200. This squirted stuff is only 100. Add the nuts and maraschino cherry and a dollop of guilt and it adds up to maybe 600. I still have 1,900 calories to go.

"Breakfast: black coffee, no calories; two slices of whole wheat toast, 110 calories; tomato juice, 50 calories; bran and skimmed milk, another 100; butter, 50. The same breakfast I always eat, and it adds up to 310 calories. No sacrifice, which leaves me 1,590. I have a sandwich for lunch. Bread, 100 calories; lettuce, maybe 5; tuna filling, 165 for water-packed; a glass of skim milk, 85. That's 358—say 400 with a cookie. That leaves me 1,190 calories for dinner. After a sundae like this, who needs a big dinner? Tonight we ate gourmet style. A shrimp cocktail, filet mignon with Bearnaise sauce, asparagus with Hollandais sauce, a baked potato and a good vintage wine."

"On a diet? I don't believe it."

"Count up the calories," Judy laughs. "The shrimp cocktail, five shrimp runs about 70 calories; the baked potato, 155; the filet, 400; the sauces, 50 each; a large serving of asparagus is 25. Altogether it adds up to 760 calories and, say, 200 more for the wine—then, for a psychological uplift, this!" She points to the sundae dish happily. "See why we call it a gourmet diet?"

"And you lose weight?" I ask astonished.

"Of course. The secret is sticking within our calorie allowance. Count them and plan your meals properly. There's very little gourmet food you can't have. Roast turkey, bouillabaise, beef Bourguignonne—get a good calorie counter and go to town."

"As for losing weight," John says seriously. "I've taken off ten pounds in the last month. Maybe that's slow, but it's better for the body than a quick loss. Each month I feel a bit younger." He carefully spooned up the last bit of ice cream. "Order another sundae and start dieting with us."

I look at the list of flavors and nod. "I think I'll just do that."

To make this type of diet work, you absolutely must have a good accurate source of calorie counts—and you must use it. Most doctors would advise against relying on this diet for an extended period of time, but the results are irrefutable—and, if you have a sweet tooth, nearly irresistible.

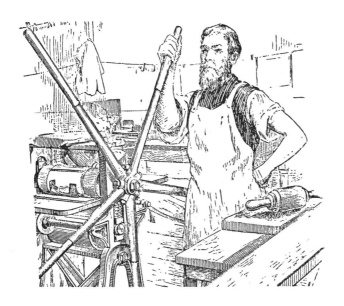

THE ANYTIME
EXERCISE PLAN

You don't have to change your routine to follow this exercise plan. In fact, you don't even have to stand up.

I met Daryl in a diner off Route 80 crossing Nebraska. We were both driving cross-country in opposite directions, I in a passenger car and Daryl in a trailer truck. We shared a booth because the diner was crowded, and we hit it off at once. When I told him I wrote for a living, he shook his head. "Now, that's one thing a trucker hardly gets to do—read."

"Even when you're off duty?"

"Even then. These crazy shifts we drive take everything out of us. Time gets to be pretty precious, and you don't like to waste it on a book." Then, seeing my face, he went on quickly, "Not that reading has to be a waste of time, it's only . . ."

"I understand."

"Well—you want the time for your family. Hey, I don't even get a chance to play ball, and I always used to be an athletic guy. I played sandlot baseball and almost made it to the big time. But since I've been trucking, I'm lucky if I get to toss a ball around with my kids."

I looked at his trim build in surprise. "You seem to be in good shape."

He smiled. "Well, that's kind of a crazy secret."

"A secret?"

Looking around first to be sure we weren't being overheard, Daryl lowered his voice. "If the other guys knew, they'd give me a hard time about it—and probably over CB radio at that. That's all I'd need!"

"But what's the secret?"

"Well—" He opened his jacket and leaned back from the table. "Look." He tensed his stomach muscles, starting at the waist and then moving upward in a sort of roll, then reversing and rolling down. Under his tight T-shirt, I could see the contractions knot and relax the muscles. After a couple of rolls, he stopped with a grin and zipped up his jacket. "I do that for more than two hours every day. Oh, not all at once, but in fifteen-minute intervals. Then I roll my shoulders and tense and relax my biceps, then my forearms. It's a little harder with my hips and legs, but I get them going, too. Tense and relax, again and again. You try that every day for two hours, and you'll have muscles like rocks!"

Fascinated, I ask, "What started you on that?"

"I guess it was my wife. You know, trucking is really a sedentary way of life. Oh yeah, I know the trucks are big and you're handling a monster out there on the road, but it's not really physical exercise. Look, I was getting a beer belly because whatever I did, I did it sitting down. My exercise was walking from the cab to a diner or a bar to hoist a few. When I got home, I didn't want to exercise any more than I wanted to read. I wanted to spend the time with my wife and kids, but I tell you, my wife didn't like it one bit—I mean all that flab."

"What did she do?"

He raised one hand. "Not what she did, but the kind of cracks she'd make, like she was kidding me ... in a loving way. It bothered me, and that's when I got onto this tension stuff, tensing my stomach muscles and relaxing them. I started there and gradually began doing it with all my muscles."

"And it worked?"

"It did—along with laying off the beer. Not right away, although I began to feel better right away. But after a few months of it, I began to feel myself hardening up. You ought to try it."

"Well, I don't do that much driving, but I'm going to do it for the rest of this trip."

I took Daryl's advice to heart, and during the next few days, I tensed and relaxed in a kind of isometric dance. I didn't have a CB, so I played local stuff on my AM radio, and found myself tensing in time to the music. What I did notice was a lot less stiffness when I'd stop for the afternoon. I wasn't as cramped as I used to be during the first half of the trip.

Later, visiting some friends, the talk turned to exercise and keeping fit. I told them about Daryl's method and how great it was for driving.

Nancy, a young housewife with three young children, nodded enthusiastically. "Your friend the trucker hasn't invented anything new. He's just rediscovered it."

"What do you mean?"

"Just that I've been doing that exact routine since my first baby was born. After I came back from the hospital, my obstetrician told me I ought to do some stomach exercises to tighten up my gut. I just couldn't get into an exercise routine, but when my slacks stopped fitting me, I hit on the tension and relaxation method. I'd do it while I was carrying the baby, cleaning the house, making dinner or doing the dishes. Even when I was rocking the baby off to sleep—we had a cradle—I'd sit there and tense as I pushed the cradle, then relax as I pulled it, I'd get into a rhythm and just let go!"

"Did it help?"

"Look for yourself." Nancy jumps up and pulls up her sweater. She's wearing slacks and a shirt, and her stomach is as flat as a board. "It's just a fantastic way of keeping yourself trim," she tells us enthusiastically. "And what's great about it is that you can do it anywhere—and at any time and right around the house. And I do it to music, too. It's almost like dancing, and you can work on any muscle you want, any muscle that's stiff or getting flabby. I do it to my glutei and it firms them up. Look." Turning, she bends forward, tensing and relaxing her buttocks. "A half hour of that a day and you look sensational in slacks."

"Now, don't overdo it, Nancy," her husband laughs.

Nodding appreciatively, I say, "You do look great in them, Nancy. I think between you and Daryl I've discovered the lazy man's perfect exercise."

"Not so lazy. It takes a lot of energy to do it. It wouldn't be an exercise if it didn't."

"You have a point there!"

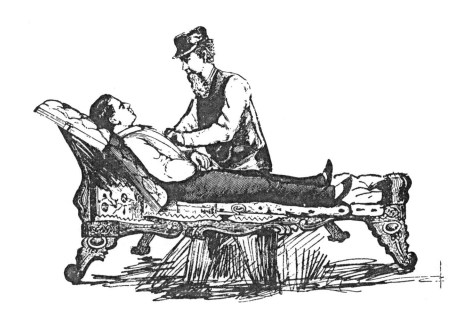

THERE'S THE RUB

Here's a technique that's almost guaranteed to bring back your enthusiasm and vigor the next time you're exhausted from a long day at work or a heavy exercise program.

"I am walking on air!" Amanda tells us. "I have just had the most glorious session with my masseuse. I don't think there's anything in the world as great as a good massage!"

"Do you really think it takes off fat?" Shirley asks uneasily. "I'm just desperate about my hips, and my friends all tell me massage is the answer."

We've met in Peter's office to discuss some unpleasant legal matters, and we are all relieved to have the conversation sidetracked.

Arnold, the doctor in the group, tells Shirley, "Massage is not the answer. Whatever Amanda says, it won't take off excess weight any more than it will get rid of your wrinkles."

"Well, what will it do?" Shirley asks.

"Make you feel great!" Amanda answers quickly. "Isn't that enough? I've never been as relaxed as I am after a massage."

"What was your massage like?" I ask her.

"My masseuse is Swedish, and she combines a sort of light stroking with a slow kneading that gets deep into the muscles. Then she does a lot of tapping and slapping—oh, I don't know. It's just good."

"What massage can do," Arnold says definitely, "is help you get rid of all the byproducts of fatigue. Say you do some heavy exercise and end up exhausted, or maybe you're exhausted after a hard day's work. Well, a good massage stimulates the circulation and helps all the fatigue toxins like lactic acid get into the perspiration and urine and out of the body.

"But the point is," he tells Shirley seriously, "it just will not take weight off, and so many people think it will. The only weight lost in massage is lost by the person giving the massage! In fact, that may be the secret. Learn to give a good massage and it will take off weight. In fact you can start with me."

"Very funny," Shirley says coolly. "But I still don't see why massage can't at least move the fat away from my hips."

Arnold looks at the ceiling for help. "Shirley! You should know better than that. Fat is living tissue in your body. You can't just massage it away. Where the hell would it go? A lot of people think that pummeling and pinching the fat will break it up an let the blood carry it away, but they just don't understand anatomy."

"Can't you massage hard enough to break up fat deposits?" Amanda asks. "I'm sure my masseuse does that."

Arnold shakes his head. "If you pressed that hard, you'd destroy the tissues and damage the body—really damage it. To tell you the truth, the unvarnished truth, if it does anything, massage puts on weight."

"What?" Amanada's eyes get round. "How?"

"How? By improving the circulation. That would bring more blood to the fatty tissue, and with the extra blood, extra nourishment that would be stored as fat. How's that for logic?"

"Well, I never heard of that!" Amanda protests.

"Oh, it's just a far-out thing. Don't consider it seriously. I just mentioned it to show how silly it is to expect miracles from massage. But I'll tell you, while we're talking about the subject and I'm giving you all this free medical advice, I'll give you a little more. Massage can be dangerous."

"How?" I ask. "I've never heard that."

"Just think about it. In the wrong hands—and I mean that literally—a massage can make a torn muscle worse or it can injure a nerve or even hurt your circulation. Say you've got a blood clot on a vessel that's near the surface. Deep massage could set it loose and cause it to float through the bloodstream. If it ends up in the heart or lungs, it might cause death."

In a frightened voice, Amanda said, "I never knew that!"

"Well—it's not a common possibility, but if you have something like thrombophlebitis, it could happen. Anyway, you should get a medical checkup before you go in for massage. Arthritics, for example, can have some painful experiences with massage. They should avoid it. And diabetics—they can be hurt if the massage is too rough. Oh, I could go on."

"You've done pretty well," Shirley says. "You've scared me off. I didn't know massage could be that dangerous."

"Oh, no," Arnold laughs. "I've just given you all the remote possibilities. Sure, you should get a medical checkup before you go in for it, but for that matter you ought to get a medical checkup before you go in for a lot of things."

"Such as?"

"Any heavy athletic sport, jogging, tennis. It's just good common sense."

"What about vibrators?" Shirley asks. "Are they good for massage?"

Arnold shrugs. "If they're too violent, like some of the

message belts in gyms, they can hurt you. They can damage your kidneys or spleen. Or if you have a bad back, stay away from them."

"But what about the little vibrators you hold in your hand? Are they good?"

"If they make you feel good, sure."

"I'm not so sure that they're good to use on the face," I put in. "Somewhere I've read that it's very easy to damage the facial muscles with the wrong kind of massage."

"The face, maybe, but I don't think they can hurt the rest of the body. They're too gentle."

Peter, who's been silently listening to all this, suddenly speaks up. "Do you know, what none of you have mentioned is the kind of massage that puts you back on your feet."

"What's that?" I ask curiously.

"Well, my girlfriend and I frequently massage each other's feet. You know, as the foot goes, so goes the head."

"What does that mean?" Amanda asks.

"It's an old Oriental saying, and it means that as long as your feet feel good, you've got a good chance to keep your head on straight. Or, you can't be comfortable when your feet hurt. So we massage each other's feet. There's a real art to it."

"Show us," I suggest.

"Let's see—take off your shoes and socks, Shirley, and I'll demonstrate." He picks up Shirley's foot and twists it gently, bending it at the ankle, inward and then out. "To start, you do that with both feet. Then you grab all the toes from above and bend them upward. Then you take each toe separately and roll it in a circle."

He suits his actions to his words and Shirley giggles. "I like it!"

"Next, you slip the fingers between the toes, bend the foot down, and pull it toward you."

"That hurts a little," Shirley says, flinching.

"Only for a moment. Now flex your toes up and down while I squeeze your foot. Got it? Good. Now I separate each toe from the next and pull it gently. Then I press each toe firmly between my thumb and index finger. Last, I push my thumb into the hollow between each bone and run it up to the ankle, like so. There. How does that feel?"

Shirley stands and takes a few steps, then turns in delight. "Why, it's great! Peter, you can massage my feet anytime."

"I think we're on to something good," Amanda says, "Let's go over that again while I take notes."

We all reach for pencils and paper, delighted to postpone our legal business a bit longer, while Peter demonstrates again, this time on Amanda, who leans back contentedly.

Because massage is so relaxing, half an hour of it before sex can give you and your partner a more satisfying sexual experieince. And some massage techniques—for many parts of the body—are so sexually stimulating they're called "erotic massage." You might want to look into these.

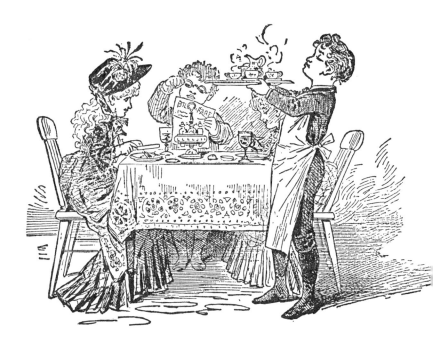

HAVE YOUR DIET
AND EAT CAKE, TOO

Have you been putting off dieting because your favorite food is high in calories? "Nutritional density" may be the right diet plan for you.

"I am an avocado freak," Letty confided sadly. "I've given up so many other fattening foods—I even cut out vanilla ice cream with Amaretto liqueur, and if you can give that up you've got to have an iron will. But avocados . . ." She shivered delicately. "How can I give up anything so scrumptious, so smooth and velvety? I eat an avocado and I'm Rima, the bird girl in the Amazon jungles! They have to be the most exquisite fruit."

"They are a fruit, aren't they?"

"Who knows. They grow on trees, I guess, but I've seen

them only on the produce shelves. They should be a fruit, though. Nothing as perfect as an avocado should be labeled a vegetable. It's too prosaic."

"Do you know," I said thoughtfully, "you can diet, lose weight, and still have the pleasure of eating avocados every day."

"How do I do it?" Letty asked, her eyes widening. "That sounds ecstatic."

"Let me see. You know, of course, that you can lose weight eating anything—even vanilla ice cream and Amaretto . . ."

"I didn't know anything of the sort! I can gain weight just looking at pictures of ice cream and avocados. Avocados have more calories per ounce than—than—I don't know. They're just plain fattening—and delicious!"

I laughed. "Yes, but you must know that all diets boil down to one thing—caloric intake."

"I guess so," Letty said slowly, "but isn't that Catch-22? I mean, big deal—all the yummy foods are high in calories."

"Ah, but suppose we drop the concept of calories and twist the dietic prism just one turn?"

"Them's pretty fancy words, but I suspect they're going to boil down to counting calories in the end."

"Yes and no. There's been a lot of research lately into the concept of nutritional density. ND."

"Nutritional density. It has a nice solid sound to it. What does it mean?"

"It's just a statistical way of looking at food. Let's say you need a certain amount of nutrients."

"Is that *you* me, or the universal *you*, like *one* needs."

"We'll make it you, Letty. You weigh about 130 pounds."

"Come on, now. It's bad enough I weigh 128. Don't push me up. The point is I must, I *absolutely* must drop over eight pounds by next weekend. I'm going out to a *very* fancy wedding and the only dress I have fit me when I was 120 pounds. Now I'm bulging out of it and I can't afford another."

"You could fast for a week?"

"I could as easily run the Boston marathon. I know what I

can and can't do. Tell me about nutritional density. I have a
strange ESP feeling that it may be the answer I'm looking for."

"Well, as a 128–pound woman, you need about 2,000
calories a day to keep your own weight, not losing or gaining.
You also need some basic nutrients, vitamins, and minerals."

"I follow. Slowly, but I follow."

"Well, avocados—rather, one avocado, supplies—oh, let's
say four units of vitamin E."

"Is that enough?" Letty asked anxiously.

"No. You should have about 12 units a day, but that's one
avocado. You don't live on one avocado a day. Other foods
give you more E. The point is, you must consider the nutrient
value of an avocado in terms of your needs—that's the
nutritional density."

"I'm not sure I'm still following, but go on."

"If you need 12 units of vitamin E each day, and an avocado
supplies you with 4—it gives you about one-third of your daily
requirement."

"I get that."

"Okay. Now an avocado has about 280 calories. If you need
2,000 a day . . ."

"But I need less. I want to lose weight."

"Fine, but first let's consider your stable weight. You neither
lose nor gain on 2,000. Now you must figure the nutritional
density of an avocado in terms of its nutritional value."

"I am defintely no longer following you!"

"Well . . . let's get back to vitamin E. An avocado supplies a
third of your daily need. Now take the caloric percentage of
the avocado."

"What the hell is that?"

"It's 280/2,000ths—14 percent."

"It is?"

"Sure. Now to find your nutritional density for vitamin E in
avocados, divide 33 by 14. It comes out about 2.4, which,
incidentally, is very good. Any density over one means you're
getting a good value—nutritionally—out of the food."

"And what about the other vitamins?"

"Oh, you can just figure a nutritional density for each, and for the minerals too, with the same method. Just divide the proportion of the nutrient each food supplies by its percentage of your daily calorie intake. Then you build your diet around avocados, or whatever."

"I'm beginning to enjoy this."

"Let's see—you still count calories," I said apologetically. "Try for 1,100 or 1,200 a day, but work in at least a half of an avocado with each meal. Just remember nutritional density."

"In what way?"

I scratched my head. "Well—shellfish, eggs, cantaloupe, raw green vegetables, Chinese bean curd, fortified cereals—all of those things have good nutritional densities. Work them into your diet."

"What you're saying is, get your money's worth, in nutrition, out of your food."

"And eat whatever you want, if it's nutritionally sound. Don't use calories as your yardstick. Use nutritional density."

"But I'll still have to count calories!"

"Nobody promised you a rose garden—you do want to lose weight."

"Desperately!"

"Then you must count. But think of all the goodies you can eat. Just proportion your calories."

"How?"

"Well, about 500 for dinner and 300 for lunch, maybe 250 for breakfast and 150 for a snack—whenever you need it. And let's see—eat about three fruits a day and make sure one's a citrus fruit. Get a lot of protein, but cut down on meat. Eat cheese and eggs and fish, lots of fish, and of course bread and skim milk—you get the picture?"

"And a very pretty picture it sounds, especially the avocados. I'm going to stop in the greengrocer on my way home and pick up five. This should be heaven!"

I met Letty a couple of weeks later, and she still looked as slim and lovely as she had before. "I'm kind of glad you didn't decide to use that diet," I told her admiringly.

"Oh, but I did." She smoothed her dress over her hips. "Can't you tell? I dropped almost ten pounds."

"And you fit into your wedding dress—I mean the dress you wanted to wear to the wedding?"

"Well . . . It was a bit loose on me, so I treated myself to a new one. After all, you don't lose ten pounds every day."

"I certainly don't."

"But one thing I have to tell you. Your diet is just like Weight Watchers. My cousin is on that, and we compared notes."

"Ah, but can she eat avocados?"

"You're right!" Her face glowed. "Now, that was heaven!"

The ND diet is based on calorie counting, but with an added twist: you also look at the nutritional value of what you eat. A "nutritionally dense" food contributes more toward your minimum daily requirements than it does toward your calorie limit for the day. Foods you might not think you could eat on a diet, such as avocado, will often have surprisingly high ND scores, so you can eat moderate amounts of them. Again, a good calorie counter is essential; so is a listing of nutrients supplied by common foods—also available at most bookstores and drugstores. Of course, you should always be sure that your diet meets your minimum daily requirements of all essential vitamins and minerals.

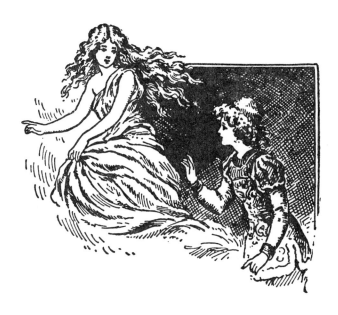

FANTASTIC SEX?
IT BEGINS IN
THE MIND

Unforgettable sex on the battlefield? Sure, with a small dose of fantasy! Here's a new kind of war story.

"When I was in the army, back in World War II," Jim tells us, "there was this fantasy going around that helped most of us get through the cold, bitter winter up in Massachusetts. We were at a staging center then, Camp Myles Standish, a dreary place with wooden barracks and mud streets and hundreds of thousands of soldiers coming and going. You spent one week in that camp and you felt that you had plumbed the absolute bottom of despair."

Jim pauses, shaking his head, and the rest of us wait. We had just finished a comfortable meal, and we were all reminiscing about the way it had been in wartime—three different wars. Jim and I were World War II veterans. Alan and Sheila, a doctor and nurse, had served in Korea, and Bill was a Vietnam vet.

Breaking the silence, Bill asks, "Was it really that bad? From all the stories I've heard about that war, it seems as if it was all fun and games."

"You know the army wasn't ever like that in any war," Jim frowns. "The trouble was, we were all just one uniform out of thousands. You could just vanish and no one would miss you."

"Tell us about the fantasy," Bill urges.

"Well, I don't know how it started, but the story was that one day a GI was hitching back from Boston. It was getting dark, and he had just about given up getting a hitch when along came this yellow convertible with a beautiful blonde driving it, a cool blonde. You know the type—shoulder-length hair, clean-cut features, a touch of the aristocrat about her— obviously rich and well-dressed. Casual, but smart.

"She stops and picks the soldier up. She doesn't say much, but she stops at a bar and buys him a few drinks instead of taking him back to camp—won't hear of his paying for them. Then she takes him back to her hotel for a wonderful night of sex.

"The next morning, she deposits him at the camp gate just in time for reveille. The soldier stumbles into line-up a little zonked out and a little ecstatic. After that, every time he hitches, he watches for her. He haunts the bar where they drank, the hotel where she stayed, always hoping to see her again—but he never does."

Jim pauses, and for a moment we're all silent. Then Bill asks, "Is that all?"

"That's all to the story, but all of us believed in that girl in the yellow convertible even while we knew it was only a fantasy. It helped us all daydream our way through the dreary hours."

"But why do you call it a fantasy?" Sheila asks. "It could be true."

I interrupt then, shaking my head. "I heard the same story—a yellow convertible and a beautiful blonde—but the army camp was Stoneman in California, and friends have told me about it happening down South and in the Midwest."

"She sure must have racked up a lot of mileage on that convertible—and wasn't there gas rationing then?" Bill laughs.

"But that's the point," Jim explains patiently. "It was just a fantasy that for some reason or other arose all over the country at almost every army base; a sexual fantasy that could set all of us daydreaming. And even though we knew it was a fantasy, we still dreamed about it. It was our sexual outlet—and man, we needed one!"

Alan, who has been listening with a smile, says, "It must have been only partly need. Sure, men and women, too, need fantasy, but beyond the need, there's the pleasure factor. We all get a kick out of fantasizing—especially on a sexual level."

Sheila says, thoughtfully, "I've always considered fantasy something—well, something to be a little afraid of. I daydreamed a lot when I was a child, and I was always told to face up to the real world—as if fantasy could somehow weaken my ability to face reality."

"I don't go along with that." Alan shakes his head. "In fact, I seem to recall reading that people with active fantasy lives have a very strong grasp on reality. Now, you take a kid who has a good, strong fantasy life, and you can bet that he'll be independent and pretty solid. From what I've read, kids who daydream make better grown-ups. I imagine that the inner worlds of delinquents are rather barren places."

We are all silent till Jim says, "What fascinates me is the sexual aspect of fantasy. Why do we get such a kick out of it when the real thing is available? I mean, I've known men who claim they can enjoy sex with their wives only when they pretend they're making love to another woman."

"Don't lay it all on the men," Bill puts in. "I just broke up with a girl who told me she couldn't make it with me unless she closed her eyes and pretended I was Burt Reynolds."

"Then the fantasy is just a crutch," Jim protests. "It's something a guy or gal needs to perform."

"I don't think that's altogether right," Sheila says thoughfully, "or altogether fair. What did you say, Alan, about deliquents' worlds being barren places without fantasy? I think that must be right. When I look at a butterfly, I fantasize myself with those gossamer wings, free and airborne—and yet I can enjoy the butterfly without my fantasy. It's the same way with sex. I can enjoy it tremendously, yet I can fantasize about it even while I'm enjoying it."

"What is your fantasy?" Alan asks.

"None of your business. You keep yours and I'll keep mine." With a little smile, Sheila takes his hand. "Intimacy is sharing, but not so completely that you know everything about me. I still have my own private places."

"Now, my sexual fantasies are no secret," Bill declares. "I fantasize that someone is watching me when I make love. Now, that really turns me on!"

A bit shocked, Jim shakes his head. "That's kinky!"

With a laugh, Bill says, "It's no big deal. Hey, some of the fantasies I've heard from other guys could curl your hair. Gals, too. I have this one girlfriend—she's hung up on Czarist Russia, and she has these sexual fantasies about being stripped and chained up by a Russian prince who forces her to do all sorts of degrading acts and ends up by violating her sexually. She claims she can get so excited with this fantasy that she has an involuntary orgasm."

Sheila makes a face. "That's a little sick, to my way of thinking."

Bill shrugs. "Different strokes for different folks. Remember, we're talking about fantasy. Anything goes."

"Perhaps," Sheila answers, "but I have a feeling that a person's fantasies must reflect the personality, like a distorting mirror. It shows you reality, but twisted a bit and altered. If the twisting is too garish, the image all askew, then the personality it reflects must be a bit weird, too."

"I don't think that's psychologically sound," Alan says. "I don't think you can set up any rules for fantasy."

"Maybe, but whatever happened to the old-fashioned sexual fantasy? When we were girls, we all dreamed of a dark, handsome man who would come into our lives—a little withdrawn, with a touch of self-torment, but alive and vital. We'd get all weak in the knees just looking at him. He was almost cruel, and he'd carry us off, sometimes against our will, but always in the end there'd be true love."

Alan says dryly, "That's not so different from the Russian prince."

"Or *The Sheik*, that crazy book from the twenties," Bill adds. "I read an old copy a few months ago, and it was a gas. This sheik kidnaps a beautiful blonde English girl and screws her until she falls madly in love with him. That was the American women's fantasy back then. They flipped when Valentino made the movie. Was that an old-fashioned sexual fantasy?"

Jim cuts in, "I know what Sheila is saying. I can stand on a street corner in the summer and watch the girls go by, watch the way their dresses cling, and I can fantasize every one in bed with me, but somehow those are—well, clean fantasies." He sighs. "I guess my own fantasies are less exotic than most, like the girl in the yellow convertible."

Alan laughs. "There's nothing so unusual about masochism in women's daydreams. I see it in a lot of my patients. I hear some wild stories about heightening their sexual pleasure by pretending that they're tied or chained during sex. There was one gal who had trouble having an orgasm. She said that once, during sex, her lover accidentally forced both her hands into a position where she couldn't free herself."

"What happened?" Sheila asks sympathetically.

"She had an instant orgasm which lasted as long as she was in that position. Don't look so shocked, honey. There's really no limit to the tricks we play with our minds to increase our pleasure."

"Alan is right," I agree. "More people than we suspect need active sexual fantasies to get a full measure of joy out of sex."

"But the point is," Alan adds seriously, "all that fantasy isn't wrong or harmful. In fact, sexual fantasy is often a very positive—to say nothing of pleasant—way of coping with a tough situation. I had a patient, a man, married to a very unattractive woman—physically unattractive. Otherwise she was a great gal. He loved her, but she just didn't turn him on sexually. Well, he overcame that with fantasy. During sex he'd fantasize the kind of woman he wanted—and he kept a very happy marriage going."

Bill says, "I still maintain, that almost all of us use fantasy for pleasure, and if the rest of you really, honestly looked into your own fantasies, you'd find some pretty far-out trips."

After a thoughtful pause, Jim answers, "Well—to be perfectly frank, I'll confess that some of my sexual fantasies are not quite as—well, ordinary as I've pretended. I should also confess," he adds quickly as the rest of us smile, "that I always feel guilty when I have them. I guess I'm a bit of a fraud, but now I'm going to think over what you all said, and maybe I'll let some of my unusual fantasies have their way."

"Since it's truth time," Bill teases, "just what were those unusual fantasies?"

Jim shakes his head. "I'm with Sheila. They're none of anyone's business but mine. I have some secret places, too, and I'm not about to show anyone else the road to them—but you know, I think now I'll walk that road a bit more often and get more pleasure out of it."

Doctors tell us that fantasizing is healthy, whether about sex or any other aspect of life. Nothing else could possibly be as private, if you choose to keep it that way. So try dreaming a little—even when you're wide-awake.

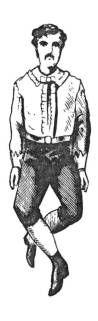

RELAXATION WITHOUT DRUGS

The tensions of modern living can sometimes seem almost overwhelming, and too many people think drugs are the best answer. I know of a better one.

"What I'm prescribing for you," Dr. Henig told my friend Irv, "is a hefty dose of Valium. Now, it may have some unpleasant side effects, like severe depression. I want you to watch out for that."

Flat on his back in bed with a very bad back, Irv took the doctor's prescription uncertainly. "But isn't that a tranquilizer, Valium? If you're just going to tranquilize me, forget it! This back is real."

With a little sigh, Dr. Henig sat down on the chair next to

the bed. "We're all victims of labeling," he explained. "Even the drug companies. Valium is a very good muscle relaxant. You're flat on your back because your muscles are all knotted up. I'm prescribing a muscle relaxant to unkink all of those muscles. It's as simple às that."

"But isn't it a tranquilizer?"

"In the sense that relaxed muscles reduce mental stress, yes. It will work as a tranquilizer. But first and foremost, it's a muscle relaxant."

In the next few days, I saw my friend make a steady, uneventful recovery. Whatever Dr. Henig claimed for Valium as a muscle relaxant, still I saw it work as a tranquilizer. Irv was much calmer than usual and accepted his week in bed philosophically. "I can't fight it, so I might as well enjoy it. There are a dozen books I want to read, and this is my chance."

Some months later, I reached a point where I felt the need to unwind, to relax completely. Work had piled up to an overwhelming load, and I could feel every muscle in my body tensing up. I thought of Irv and Dr. Henig's little talk about Valium, and I wondered if that wasn't exactly what I needed.

"I don't think so," Irv said thoughtfully when I mentioned it to him. "Why don't you do what I'm doing now?"

"What's that?"

"Yoga."

"Come on! I ask you about a tranquilizer, and you talk to me about yoga?"

"Well, sure. It makes sense if you understand what yoga is. I've been doing it ever since my bad back attack. Basically, it's one of the best—and incidentally the oldest—ways of relaxing your body and your mind."

"How can it do that?"

"By doing just what Dr. Henig told me Valium did. It relaxes your body first and unravels all the tension and muscle knots. Inevitably your mind follows along, and you gradually unwind all over. I tell you what—come along with me tonight to my yoga class, and you'll see what I mean."

I agreed reluctantly; I had always lumped yoga with

astrology and all the mystical nonsense that clutters up our civilization. But I was just physically uncomfortable enough to give it a try—at least before I tried Valium.

My reluctance at the beginning of the evening turned into grudging admiration for the method before the session was over, and within a month I had joined a yoga class myself and was experiencing, firsthand, that delightful "unraveling" Irv had told me about.

The first exercise I was shown that evening was extremely simple. I was told to simply lie down on my back or stomach and go limp. I was to think of every muscle in my body, from scalp to toe, and as I thought of each one, to try to relax it.

Breathing, the instructor told me, is a very important part of yoga. "Try this very simple routine. Sit down comfortably and close one nostril with a finger. Now breathe through the other, slowly, deeply and with your mouth closed. Then switch nostrils."

Doing this, I was suddenly conscious of the actual act of breathing, something I had taken for granted all my life. I could feel my chest expand, my lungs fill, the air travel through my nasal passages, and almost—it seemed—the oxygen enter my blood!

Ridiculous? Perhaps, but the sense was there. I did another breathing exercise, lying on my back with my knees bent, inhaling and exhaling only with my abdomen, feeling it swell under my fingertips, and again feeling the curious consciousness; something I can describe only as a sudden understanding of my body and its physical processes.

I found the same understanding in the exercises to relax my eyes and neck. For the eyes, I would look up for five seconds, then to the left, close them, then, opening them, look to the right and then down.

With my neck, it was a simple roll. I would drop my head forward for a few seconds. Then, taking a deep breath, I'd let my head roll around until I was back to my original position, chin on my upper chest. I had never realized how tense and spastic those neck muscles were. I could feel them stretching painfully the first few times, then more easily. But surely, I thought, I use these muscles every day. Why is it only now when I stretch them out that I feel how tense and knotted they are?

It was the same with my feet. I would stand on my toes, then roll onto the outer edges of my feet, back to the heels, then the inner edges and back to my toes—stretching and unkinking muscles I was hardly aware of before.

For leg stretching I would sit on the floor mat, my legs outstretched and wide apart. I'd bring my arms way up over my head, then come forward till I reached one of my feet, my head at my knee. I'd hold that position to the count of ten, then repeat it with my other foot.

Another, slightly more arduous exercise, started with me on my back, my hands at my sides. Then I would slowly lift my legs, up, up and over, until they touched the floor behind my head. Again, muscles I had never been aware of all up and down my back stretched and pulled and unknotted as I moved.

In another exercise, I would lie on my stomach, bend my knees, and reach back to grab my ankles. Then, arching my back, I would rock back and forth slowly. In this routine, the muscles of my abdomen and shoulders would be stretched. Oddly enough, stretching seems to go hand-in-hand with relaxing. As the knots and kinks are pulled out, the muscle becomes better able to contract normally, to end up in a relaxed state.

"The exercises in yoga," the instructor told us in the beginning, "are numerous, but you must start simply—start, in fact, with those exercises that don't even seem exercises—the breathing and body twisting, rotating the head, and rolling on your feet—then slowly you must work up to headstands and the more difficult positions. You'll notice that I didn't even suggest to the beginners that they try the lotus position. That comes much later when all your muscles are stretched and relaxed."

Later, too, I found, comes an exercising of the senses. Through meditation we were taught how to stretch and relax our minds. Visually, we became aware of colors and patterns, acoustically, of noises and sounds, repetitive and pleasant sound, from classical music to dripping water. Touch, smell, taste—all the senses were exercised, and we were taught to use them all to relax.

It all came tantalizingly close to mysticism, but I went along with it for curiosity's sake. Still, for my part, the physical relaxation, the stretching and loosening of the body muscles, even in an exercise as simple as the head roll, was the most intriguing part of yoga.

"I can see now why you don't need a drug to relax," I told Irv after the first two months.

He reached out quickly and rapped the wooden table we were sitting at. "Knock wood, I hope I never do again. Maybe yoga's the answer, but even if it's not, I enjoy it and, best of all, it doesn't depress me."

> *Yoga's natural approach is what makes it so valuable an exercise program. Instead of masking the symptoms of tension, yoga corrects its cause: the wound-up state of mind that brings on the physical problems.*

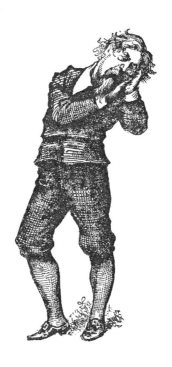

EXERCISE FOR PEOPLE WHO CAN'T

Suppose you want to exercise, but have a physical disability—arthritis, for example. You shouldn't let that get in the way. Even if you can't do regular exercise, there is probably a special exercise program that's right for you.

In the late afternoon, Annie's living room is a pleasant blend of lavender and gray. The lamps glow softly, and the drawn drapes hide the driving rain outside. I sip my tea contentedly. "Tea in the afternoon was a magnificent idea."

Annie shrugs. "As long as we had some business and you were willing to come here . . . Why not be civilized. We tend to forget the amenities."

I nod, glancing curiously at her hands as she poured another cup of tea. "You do that so easily."

She laughs and pushes back her short gray hair. "So you remember my arthritis."

"How could I forget? Last year you were in such pain."

Annie gestures toward the windows. "In this kind of weather, it still isn't good, but it's far, far better than it was. Part of it is medication, but a big part is my exercise."

Frowning, I say, "But last year you told me that you couldn't exercise. We were all talking about how necessary exercise is at our age, and you said . . ."

"I know," she smiles. "I remember exactly. I said, 'Except for an arthritic.' We can't exercise because it's too painful, but unless we do, we get stiffer and stiffer. It's the Catch-22 of arthritis."

"But you say you have been exercising."

Annie lifts her teacup and sips, then replaces it carefully on the lacquered table between us. "I couldn't do that last year. The fine motions were too much for me, or if I could do it, it hurt. That's what's so miserable about arthritis—the hurt."

"And now?"

"Oh, it still hurts, but not the same way. I kept looking for some way around Catch-22, and for a while I thought swimming was the answer."

"In this weather?"

"I joined a health club, and they had a good-sized indoor pool. I never used the gym." She shrugs. "Just the thought of working out with my joints terrified me, but the pool was something else. I got into a routine three days a week, and I built up to six laps. It was the only exercise I've been able to do in years."

"Did it help?"

Annie leans back with a frown. "Yes and no. It did seem to make me feel better, but it was such an effort getting over there—and expensive. I live on a pretty tight budget, and health clubs keep upping their prices. Then, too, when the weather is bad, I have to take cabs." She shakes her head. "It all began to get out of hand, and to tell you the truth, I wondered if the good results were worth the tension involved. Arthritis is affected by tension, you know."

I nod. "But you do seem improved."

"Ah, but that's not the swimming. I have a niece who's an occupational therapist, and she came for a visit and was terribly upset by how limited my life was. She told me I must exercise, and when I explained Catch-22 to her—that the more exercise I did, the harder it was to exercise—she just shook her head in disgust. 'Aunt Annie,' she told me, 'you had the wrong advice. Now I'm going to give you a set of exercises that I want you to stay with faithfully, and we'll see what happens.' "

I knew Annie's niece and I smiled at the imitation. "Did they work?"

"Well, look at me!" She puts her teacup down and spreads her arms, stands up, bends and then straightens. *"Voilà!* No pain. I just couldn't do that last year."

Fascinated, I ask, "Tell me about the exercises."

"Well—they're so mild, so gentle, that you don't really think of them as exercises. I guess that's just the point—a different concept of motion. They're so easy that you feel no pulling or stretching or pain—and yet they do work. Over a period of time, your muscles loosen up and your joints become freer. You see, with arthritis—at least with rheumatoid arthritis, the type I have—the crippling effect of the disease works on the bones. The bones become so painful that you don't want to move them, and the lack of motion aggravates the condition. Your circulation suffers and your muscles suffer."

"And these exercises?"

"Well, look. Here's the first one. I do this sitting down in a regular chair." Annie perches on the edge of a straight-backed chair, her head held erect, drops her head to her chest, then lifts it. "See? That's all there is to that one. I do it five times. In fact, I do each exercise five times."

"Just bending your head forward and lifting it? Why, that's no exercise at all."

"Correction. That's a very, very gentle exercise. In the next one I drop my head to the right, then to the left. Then I turn to the left, trying to touch my shoulder with my chin, then to the right. Each motion five times, and so much for the head."

There is exercise here, I realize as I watch Annie, but a slow, gentle sort of exercise. All the joints of the neck are moved.

The next motion exercises her trunk. She holds her arms out and twists to the right, then to the left; then, hands on hips, she bends to the left and to the right. Breathing in, she lifts her arms, and breathing out, she drops them, bending toward the floor.

Next come the legs. All Annie does is straighten each leg. Then with her knees slightly apart and her feet off the floor, she turns her feet in and out, exercising the ankle joints.

"That's the sitting part," Annie tells me cheerfully. "Let me show you the rest. It's lucky I'm wearing pants!"

She stretches out on her back on the living-room rug, her arms at her side, raises her arms over her head, then back to her side. Then, keeping her palms up, her arms on the rug, she moves her arms in big swings from above her head to her side.

"I love this one because it takes me back to when I was a kid. We used to do this in the clean snow and call it making butterflies. God! How limber I was then."

Annie clasps her hands behind her head and brings her elbows together, then apart. Her shoulder joints have been thoroughly exercised, and now she goes to the elbows. First she holds her arms straight at her sides. Then she brings her hands to her shoulders and straightens them. Then she moves her forearms from her side to her stomach, exercising the elbow joint in another direction.

Then the wrists. With her elbows bent, she turns the palms toward her face, then out, then makes a fist, straightens the fingers, separates them, and wiggles them. All the joints of the hand have been moved.

Next comes her spinal column. She stretches her arms forward and pulls her head and shoulders off the rug, then brings each knee to her chest. Her hips are being moved as she stretches each leg as far to the side as it will comfortably go. Then, with her arms flat on the rug, she pulls her feet forward toward her face, then away, flexing the ankle joints.

Without a pause, Annie rolls on her side, and, keeping her knees straight, raises her top leg, then repeats it on the other side.

Her last exercise is to roll on her stomach and first raise her head and stomach, then, bending her knees, lift each thigh in turn. Finally, knees still bent, she lets her lower legs fall to each side. Each motion, from beginning to end, is done five times.

Finally she gets to her feet very easily and grins. "And that's the second time today. I think I deserve another biscuit."

"But those exercises aren't enough to take off weight . . ."

"Heavens no! I'm just rewarding myself for doing them, not making up for lost calories. In fact, I think I'll have a chocolate biscuit, too."

"The thing that impresses me," I tell her, "is that every joint in your body was moved."

"Exactly, and not strenuously, and without weight on it. The point is, even badly crippled arthritics can do these, at least once and maybe work up to five times. I don't do more than five because then Catch-22 sets in and I lose more by exerting myself than I gain in mobility. That's the key point, mobility. This has increased my mobility tremendously—and of course decreased some of the pain. Not all, but some." She looks at the windows and sighs. "Except on a rainy day like this."

"Well, you had that extra biscuit as a reward. I'll have one for the rain. They're very good biscuits."

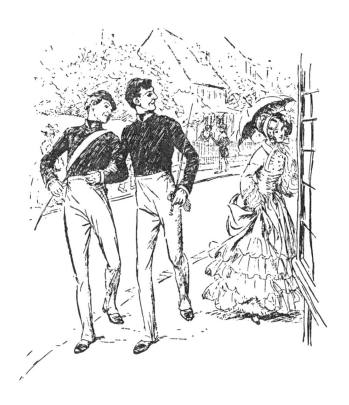

THE UNKNOWN LOVER

Mix mystery and sex and what do you get? Sexual excitement par excellence!

"The most exciting sexual encounter I ever had," Tommy said, "was with someone whose name I never learned."

Helen sipped her drink and raised one carefully plucked eyebrow. "I didn't know you were that quick with women, Tommy," she murmured with a brittle edge to her voice.

The four of us were sitting on the back deck of Irv's summer house at the beach. It was a lovely August evening, the cool ocean wind blowing away the last of the day's heat, and the low sun streaking the Pacific sky with pale pastels. We had been talking of love and sex, and Irv had just finished a very tender story of a love affair during the Vietnam war.

"I'm not anything with women," Tommy drawled lazily. "You know I'm gay. I'm talking about a man. We met on the street—if you'll believe it—I guess you could call it a classic pickup—and I took him up to my apartment."

"Wasn't that dangerous?" Irv asked mildly. "I mean, taking someone you didn't know into your house like that?"

"I'm a very big boy," Tommy said dryly. "I'm six-three in my stockinged feet, and my friend for the evening was short and frail—anyway, give me credit for judging personality."

"Before you even knew his name?" Helen asked.

"Why not? Anyway, the point is, there was no danger. He came up with me, and we had sex, and it was fantastic. Just wonderful."

Puzzled, I say, "But from what I know, and from everything I've ever read, that kind of anonymous sex can't be—well, there's no intimacy, no sharing. It's all physical!"

"Don't knock 'all physical.' Don't you see, the very anonymity of the whole thing makes it all the more exciting—even easier."

"Easier how?" Helen asks, frowning.

"Well, it's a matter of risk. With someone you know, a friend, you're taking a chance when you get into a sexual relationship, homosexual or heterosexual. If it doesn't work out, you're stuck with the commitment. You have something to lose. That can keep you on edge, anxious. I know people who are so scared of a relationship and all it entails that they avoid sex altogether."

"But aren't you doing just the opposite?" I asked. "Aren't you avoiding a relationship altogether in favor of sex?"

"Exactly. You hit it on the head. And by avoiding the relationship, I can relax in the sexual part of it all."

"You know," Irv said slowly. "Tommy isn't so far out. I'm single and heterosexual . . ."

"Well, bully for you!" Tommy leaned back with a smile.

"No, let's be serious. I say that only because so often you

guys are accused of having anonymous sex because you're gay. But I've had it on the heterosexual level."

"Do tell! Maybe that's what's wrong with us." Helen's smile seemed a little forced, and I became aware that her weekend with Irv hasn't been completely perfect.

Irv reached out and took her hand. "Now, don't get uptight. We've got a good thing going—we just have to work at it. Nothing good comes easy."

"That's a really original cliché!" Helen murmured, pulling back her hand.

"Tell us about your anonymous sex," I asked quickly.

"If you can stand another wartime story."

Tommy groaned, but I said, "Don't mind him. Tell us."

"Well, I was on furlough and I was taking a bus home—one of those long night runs. I picked a seat near the back so I could doze in private. It wasn't a crowded bus—in fact, it was almost empty—and I was just settling down when this really lovely-looking girl got on. Short dark hair and slim, and I remember her eyes—even in that darkened bus. They seemed to shine.

"She walked down the aisle past me, and I swear to God, the vibes went out. I looked back and caught her eye, and we locked glances and held them just a bit too long."

"What do you mean, too long?" Helen asked.

"Well, you know. There's a moral looking time for that sort of thing, and we looked beyond it. I smiled and she sort of looked me up and down, then walked back to my seat and said, 'Is this seat taken?' nodding at the seat next to mine.

"That fascinated me. Maybe five people in the whole bus, and she asks is this seat taken. I had to come back with something cute, so I said, 'Now it is. Sit down.'

"She had just gotten settled when the lights went out and we took off. It was a freeway run, and you could sense everyone settling in for the night. I asked, 'Where are you heading?' and she gave a big sigh and said, 'Look, soldier. I don't feel like talking. Okay?'

"I thought that was a rebuff, so I said, 'Fine,' and turned

toward the window, and then damned if she didn't reach out and put her hand on my leg and say, very softly, 'Don't get sore.'

"I put my hand on hers, and that started it."

"Started what?" I asked.

"The most exciting sexual experience I've ever had," Irv said slowly. "We began fondling each other with our hands at first. Then we kissed, and one thing led to another."

"In a bus!" Helen exclaimed.

"Well, that was just it. You see, what Tommy said about anonymity hit home. We didn't know each other, and we had nothing to lose—absolutely nothing. We both knew we'd walk away at the end of that ride, and we'd never see each other again."

"Didn't you want to?" I asked, "Especially if it was so good."

"No. The idea that we'd be strangers—that we wouldn't even know each other's name—was what freed all our inhibitions. Can't you understand that?"

"I can't!" Helen said. "It sounds perverted to me."

"Oh, come off it, Helen " Tommy said disgustedly.

But suddenly a memory stirred in me. "Now, wait a minute. I know what Irv means, and I can back him up."

"You?" Helen said, raising her eyebrows. "Now I'm shocked."

"Well, it's a war story, too—World War II—and I was stationed near Boston. I was just a kid, and I thought I was pretty hot stuff in my uniform—I think I had just gotten my corporal's stripes. Three of us went into town to pick up girls."

"They did that way back then?" Tommy murmured.

"Don't be a smart-ass. You know, I came from a pretty protected family and I had never picked up a girl in my life. But the uniform, the war—we cruised Scollay Square, and sure enough we found three girls. It didn't get to sex, but it was what we used to call a dry run. Everything but—and we never told each other our names!"

I shook my head, remembering. "The thing is, there was

that same freedom Irv and Tommy spoke of. It freed me to do things I'd never dream of doing with a girl I knew—and it freed the girl."

"And you think it was better than sex with someone you know?" Helen asked.

"Better? No, not for me, but it was for some of the other men. The point is, it was freer, and exciting. That extra bit— we'd never meet again and who gave a damn, made all the difference—and that was before the sexual revolution!"

"It's the anonymity," Tommy said. "I can see Irv's point about the dark. That's even better. No responsibilities, no recriminations. If I do something you don't like—so what? If you do something that offends me—who cares? We are ships that pass in the night."

Helen shivered. "I never could—but I can almost understand what you mean."

"Love with the anonymous stranger," Irv said. "I recommend it."

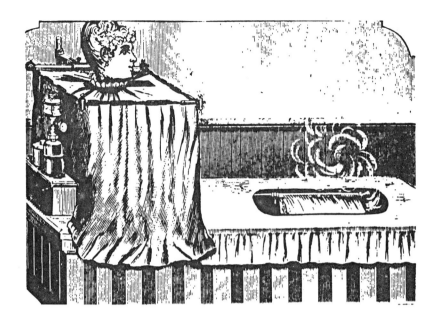

STEAM YOUR TROUBLES AWAY

A few minutes in a steam room can drain away your tensions and leave you feeling ready to take on the world.

"I think there's something ethnic about the whole thing," Sid said to me as a group of us sat side by side on the tiled seat of the steam room. We had all worked out in the gym, showered briefly, and now we were relaxing in clouds of steam, easing the knots out of our tired stomachs.

"Ethnic about what?" I asked.

"About steam. I love it. Unwinding in one of these steam rooms is my idea of the most. I can feel all the tension draining out. I'm like a tight, coiled spring winding down!"

"Just don't come to a full stop," I cautioned. "But I don't get your ethnic."

"Well, I think it's in my background, my Lower East Side Jewish background, this love of steam. I remember my father and my grandfather going to the *schvitz* baths downtown when I was just a kid. I always wanted to go along and finally, when I was a teen-ager, my dad took me. I loved it on sight!"

Shaun, on my other side, said, "Why does it have to be ethnic? I'm Irish, for God's sake—grew up in the old country and didn't come over until I was fourteen. And I love the steam room, too."

"When did you first go?"

"It was in the army." He nodded. "Yes, a gang of us had gone out on the town—in Paris on leave. We were stationed in Germany. Man, I got a head on me that night, like an enormous balloon, expanding and contracting. My first sergeant said, 'Lad, there's only one cure for you,' and he took me to this Turkish bath—a real Turkish bath!"

"Did it cure you?"

"That it did, but I still can't forget the wonder of it."

"The wonder? Come on—"

"I mean it. It was nothing like the baths in this country. It was an enormous place, tiled and all sorts of colors, filled with pillars with seats around their bases, and up above they curved into vast, tiled arches. It was like walking into a fairy-tale palace, but filled with steam so that you caught only glimpses of the arches and vaulted ceilings. Remember, I was still half-drunk, and I didn't know but that I'd walked into a dream."

"And you liked the steam?"

"I don't know which I liked most, the steam or the tiled inside of that place. I know I sat down on the base of one of the columns and breathed in that steam. I could feel my whole body straightening out, all the poisons oozing out of me. That was the beginning of my love affair with steam."

The rest of us laugh, and Al says, "Aside from everything else—I mean aside from how good it feels to spend time in a steam room—there's the health angle. You come out of a steam room, and your skin is clean, your circulation is better, and you've gotten rid of all the poisons and wastes in your system.

The rest of you can take the steam for romantic or ethnic reasons—me, I take it for health."

I lean across to Barney, the doctor in our group, and I ask, "Is all that true, about health and steam?"

Barney looks surprised. "Why ask me?"

"You're a doctor."

"I'm a gynecologist."

"Come on, you studied medicine. You should know."

"Well—I'll tell you this. If you have a heart condition or high blood pressure, the steam is no good for you."

"But if you're in good health?"

"Okay, you take the average good steam room, the temperature should be about 120 to 140 degrees."

"I thought it ran 200," Sid says, surprised.

"That's okay for a sauna where the heat is dry. With wet heat, you have to have a lower temperature for it to work well. You know, the normal skin temperature is 92, and when the steam jacks it up—even higher than the body temperature of 98 or 99—the body goes to work to try and even things out."

"How?"

"Well, for one thing the heart works harder while the skin gets rid of carbon dioxide and takes in oxygen. The body begins to sweat to try and cool the skin, and that sweat washes out all the junk that clogs your pores, the old oil and wax—at least, that's the theory behind the benefits of steam. Me, I think it's as much psychological as physical."

"Can't you get the same effects out of a hot bath?" Al asks.

"Sure, but not as subtly. In a steam bath, the temperature rises slowly. The body gets used to it. There isn't the same strain on the system—on the heart, too—as there is when you put your whole body into a hot tub. The sudden heat of the tub against the skin can break little capillaries and give those red spiders my women patients are always complaining about. Then, too, the wet steam is also supposed to be good for respiratory troubles."

"Supposed to be?" Sid asks, surprised. "I thought it definitely was."

"I don't think there's any hard evidence that it is. We all

know that steam is supposed to help people with breathing problems. You've all got kids, and you all must have used vaporizers with them when they had colds." Barney gestures around the steam room. "Essentially, this is one big vaporizer. It helps us clean out our nasal passages and lungs."

"So all in all there's a lot good about steam rooms and not much bad," Al says.

"Provided you're in good health," Barney adds. "And also provided that you replace the water your body loses when you sweat."

"So you drink a few glasses of water afterward."

"That's not enough. You lose a lot of minerals if you sweat a lot—sodium and potassium. Orange juice is good, or you can eat a banana with the water you drink. Or try a good mineral water."

"What's a good one?" I ask.

"Read the label and be sure it has potassium and sodium. But the big thing is not to overdo it." He stands up and stretches. "Like I've been in here ten minutes, and that's enough for me."

"I could spend the whole day here," Sid says, getting up reluctantly.

"Don't try it. Ten minutes is plenty."

"What I like to do," Sid says as we head for the showers, "is rub oil into my hair before I go into the steam room. It keeps my scalp in good shape, and I swear, the wet heat has some effect on the oil. When I shampoo it, my hair comes out *fantastic.*"

"I wish I had the hair to try it," Shaun sighs.

Later, over a cup of coffee, Barney says, "You know, when Shaun talked about his Turkish bath in Paris, it reminded me of one I went to in Istanbul."

"A real Turkish bath! Hey, what was it like?" Sid asks.

"Well, the steam room was a little like the one Shaun described. It was sort of cross-shaped with a high dome, and there were glass windows in the dome, blue and green and amber. The walls were marble instead of tile, and there were marble fountains with water splashing. I remember the light from the windows up high filtering through the steam in all sorts of crazy colored patterns. It was great fun."

"Did you just relax in the steam?"

"They don't let you relax. They have attendants—great big husky Turks who really work you over—pummeling and massaging you, splashing water on you and soaping you up, then washing you off. They even walk up and down on your spine—but man, they know their business. When they're finished, you really feel like a million bucks. I've never had such good results—in terms of my back. It felt great for a week afterward."

He shakes his head. "But the crazy thing about it all, the really far-out thing, was the towels."

"What do you mean?" Sid asks.

"Well, you know the crummy hotel towels we get here at the health club. They're worn and thin, and half the time they don't go around you—especially if you've got a belly like mine. Those towels in Istanbul were something else, so deep and rich and soft and big—I remember those towels more than anything else on the whole trip."

There's a moment's envious silence, and then Sid shakes his head. "Why shouldn't you? They were real Turkish towels—that's the whole point!"

"Only in Istanbul!" Barney sighs.

How to get the best of both worlds: Bring your own Turkish towels to your health club steam room.

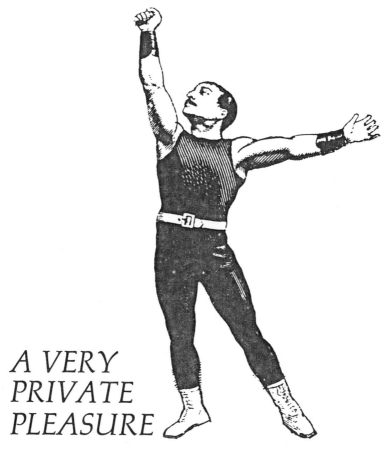

A VERY PRIVATE PLEASURE

A secret exercise technique helped one friend of mine stay fit. Even though he revealed it to me, his technique is still known only to a select few. If you try it and like it, it's up to you whether to keep it secret, too.

It's a pleasant, cool day in late summer, and my friend Neil and I have hiked up into the mountains for a day's climb. After an hour, I call a halt. "We've got to rest. I'm bushed."

Neil squats and smiles at me. "The trouble is, you're flabby. You need more exercise to keep in shape."

I look at his slim, athletic body enviously. "How do you do it? You're not even breathing hard, and I'm completely pooped."

"Exercise," he shrugs. "That's all it is."

But there's something evasive about his answer, and that afternoon when we've finished hiking and are sitting on the back porch with drinks, I bring the subject up again. "Do you belong to a gym, Neil?"

"Oh, no."

"Tennis?" When he shakes his head, I pursue my questioning. "Jogging? Bicycling?" I run down all the list of exercises I know as Neil's grin grows broader.

"What I will say," he finally tells me, "is that I enjoy my exercise out of all proportion to the good it does."

"What do you mean?"

"Well, generally when you do something that's good for you, like exercise, it's something of a chore. I've tried jogging and biking, but I've always had to force myself to do them. It got to the point where I'd wake up and look out the window, and if it was raining, I'd breathe a sigh of relief."

He laughs. "I tell you. When things get to that point, you know you're doing something wrong. There was just no pleasure in exercising. It was a drag, and I had to admit I hated it."

"Then why do it?"

"Because I hated the flab I put on without exercise even more, and besides, the exercise was a physical pleasure."

"I don't get that."

"What it did to me physically. It toned up my entire body. I felt great, but the price I had to pay for feeling great was too much."

"Now I'm confused," I say. "Are you trying to tell me that you don't exercise?"

"I don't go in for any of the 'keep busy' exercises, the jogging and biking, or the trendy exercises like tennis."

"Then what do you do?"

Neil gets a very funny look on his face and sips his drink slowly. "You've boxed me into a corner. I happen to have a secret exercise, and it's truly a secret. I've never confessed it to anyone."

Intrigued, I ask, "But you'll tell me, won't you?"

He sighs. "I don't see how I can avoid it now. The truth is—I've been a frustrated ballet dancer all my life, a real balletomaniac."

"Ballet?" I'm completely surprised.

"That's right. I've never had any formal training—in fact, I've never had any training at all. I'm much too self-conscious to take lessons, and I'm not sure I want to. It would become tedious then. As it is, I've read books on ballet. I learned the steps from the books, and I practice every morning—but I don't call it practice."

He frowns a little. "I don't know how to explain this. I guess it's just a matter of fantasy, but I begin my ballet routine, and suddenly it's as if I'm on a stage and I can hear the audience, the music—see the footlights and spots—and completely forget myself in the spell of the dance."

"Are you good at it?" I ask, fascinated. "Would you really like to try out for some professional company someday?"

Neil waves this suggestion aside impatiently. "I don't want any of that nonsense. I'm not stagestruck. I don't want to be a professional. Look, this is something I choose for pleasure—the pleasure it gives my body—and you'd better believe that ballet is the hardest, most grueling exercise there is—but also for the pleasure it gives me to do it.

"The moment it becomes a professional thing, when I have to practice so many hours a day and live up to a definite standard, it would lose all its pleasure. No, I want no part of professional dancing. I get my jollies by practicing ballet steps myself, alone in the privacy of my room—and daydreaming. In my daydreams I'm anyone. Who the hell is Rudolf Nureyev? Once I get going I can outdance him and Baryshnikov together—in any ballet.

"But even above the daydreaming, the fantasy-land, the very act of dancing gives me pleasure and it doesn't matter how well I dance nor how professionally. Sometimes I'll work out for over an hour, and it's never a chore even when I end up covered with sweat. It's something I always look forward to, always enjoy. In fact there are times at work, especially during those long, dreary business conferences, when I close my eyes and imagine I'm dancing—and that's a pleasure, too!"

"But how did this all start," I ask. "To begin with it's unusual for a man to want to do ballet. I mean—"

"Yes, I know what you mean." There's a touch of bitterness in Neil's voice. "My father was like that, too. I remember when I was ten years old, back in Columbus, Ohio, my mother took me to see a ballet and I was stunned. I had never seen such grace, such poetry. It was like liquid gold, each movement flowing into another. I just sat there with my mouth open, and afterward my head was in a whirl. All I could think of was ballet. All I could eat and sleep and dream was ballet."

Neil pauses. After a moment, I ask, "What happened?"

"My father happened," he says flatly. "He put a stop to that 'queer' nonsense. He told me straight out: ballet dancers weren't real men, and no son of his was going to get mixed up with them. I was to forget it, never to talk about it again."

"Did you?"

"I became a closet balletomaniac. I read everything I could in secret. I saved my money and whenever possible I sneaked out to see what I could, and as a result it was never more than a deep, secret yearning."

"What changed it?"

Neil shrugs. "When I left home, it was different. I could see as much ballet as I wanted, but it was too late to do anything about my own desire to dance—at least, that's what I thought. But then one summer, on a tour, I shared a room with a professional dancer on vacation.

"I was impressed by his dedication and the fact that even on vacation he practiced for a couple of hours every day. When I told him about myself and my ballet craze, he said, 'Why don't you dance?' 'Professionally?' I asked, and he said, 'No. It's too late in life for that, but do it for fun. Put on a record and dance. Pick up the steps from any basic book on ballet, and dance for the joy of it.' It was as simple as that."

Smiling a little, I ask, "Was that ballet dancer what your father thought?"

Neil shrugs. "I don't know and I don't care. I know what I

am, and that's what matters. As for a *manly* art, have you any idea of the energy it takes to dance professionally? Of the strength? For sheer strength, I'd match a ballet dancer against a football player any day. For muscular development—it's the greatest, and the most fun!"

Fascinated, I ask, "Would you dance for me?"

"No way!" Neil says emphatically. "That's a very private pleasure, a very, very private thing."

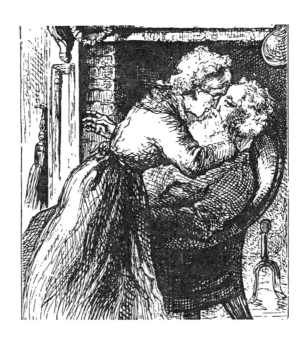

LIKE VINTAGE WINE

Have stable marriages become outdated? Not at all! A good marriage can be a source of comfort and happiness and freedom, according to six people who ought to know.

"An old love is the best," Barbara confided. "It's a little like vintage wine. Sometimes it's soft and warm and mellow. Occasionally it's corky—at times it can be downright sour—but overall, it stands the test of time."

We were sitting around the fireplace, a group of us, on one of those gray, rain-swept afternoons where the very misery of the weather drains all your energy. We had been talking idly of old and new love, and in the end we were surprised to discover that the six of us—three couples—had clocked close to a hundred years of marriage among us.

"Why do you think our marriages have lasted?" Milt asked curiously, and Barbara had countered with her comparison of old love and vintage wine. I thought about it for a moment, then said, "Yes, it sounds nice but there has to be a reason. I find it hard to believe we're all doing something right. Maybe it's sheer luck."

Cal said, "Luck—maybe. Inertia? The terrible feeling that you might break up an old marriage only to get into a new one just as bad."

"Has ours been that bad?" his wife Jessie asked, smiling. "Have you been afraid to leave it because the next might be terrible, too?"

"I wasn't talking about our marriage," Cal gestures lazily. "That's not the reason we've stayed together."

"Why have we then?"

He thought for a moment, then said, "To be perfectly honest, it hasn't been all roses, but a lot of it—most of it, in fact—has been great. But staying together—well, I think it's because we have so much in common."

"Such as?" Jessie asks, still smiling.

"The kids, our house, the boat—God, how could we ever split that up? It's more than just owning it. It's all the wonderful times we've had on it, alone on the water, just the two of us. I could never be that comfortable with anyone else."

"I think," Barbara says slowly, "that comfort is a tremendous part of it."

"How do you mean?"

"The comfort you have with a husband—or a wife. After all those years, it's just too much to lose."

Milt says, "But that doesn't follow. I know so many men who can't stand just that comfort. They feel that a marriage gets boring when you get that comfortable with your partner. There's nothing new to discover, no variety. You know each other too well."

"But that's just where the newness and variety comes in," Barbara protests.

"I don't see that."

"Well, sure it can grow dull and boring if you know the person too well and there's nothing new, nothing different. But I never find marriage dull because both of us have grown and changed in our marriage and I find that there's always something new to discover in each other."

Nodding, I say, "Yes, and a part of that is that in the right kind of marriage you never reveal yourself completely. There's always something to discover and find out about your partner."

Sally, Milt's wife, says, "You can turn it around and look at it from the other side. Once you know a person that well, you can be completely comfortable in his or her presence."

"So?"

"So you can be free to do the things you'd never do with a stranger, oh, little comfortable things, like breaking wind or belching or scratching yourself—all those things. Physically, after all these years, I'm completely at ease with my husband in a way I never could be with a new lover. So I'm fat here and there, or I have a scar or a blemish. He knows it as well as he knows his own body—and I know his."

"I still don't get it." Cal shakes his head.

"Don't you? We're so comfortable with each other that we're free to bellyache and complain and tell each other our troubles. I can groan when I get out of a chair, and during sex I can complain if he's too heavy. I can tell him to shift his weight, and I can tell him if I didn't have an orgasm or if I want another. Who needs to pretend? I know him so well, and I know he'll tell me if he's tired, or eager for sex or—or anything!"

"I think I see," Jesse says. "If you're that free, you can go a step further—"

"Exactly. You can experiment within the marriage, and it doesn't have to be the frantic kind of sexual experimenting we read about, the sort of desperate effort to find something new and different."

She hesitates a minute, then goes on. "If we experiment and it doesn't work out, okay. We can laugh at it. If it works out, that's great. We can enjoy it, or if one of us doesn't want to experiment, we can say so. The thing is, we're both so comfortable with each other that nothing is tense or anxious."

"I agree," Cal says, frowning a little. "I remember a few years ago I had an episode of impotence. We worked it out very quickly because neither of us were hung up on performance. If it didn't work out one night, what the hell—there were plenty of other nights ahead. But I talked to a friend of mine who left his wife and moved in with another woman. He split up with the second woman within a month, and it was over impotence. We all have it from time to time, but how can you work it out in the heat of proving a new relationship?"

"How can you work any problem out," Jesse says. "It all needs time. Even the nonsexual parts of marriage, where we go and who we see. I can tell Cal, 'Let's not see the Smiths because I can't stand her tonight.' He knows me well enough to realize it's a temporary thing, and he'll go along with it—but that all comes from the comfort of all those years of marriage."

"Like you said," Cal smiles at Barbara. "Vintage wine. I'll drink to that."

We all raise our glasses in silent agreement.

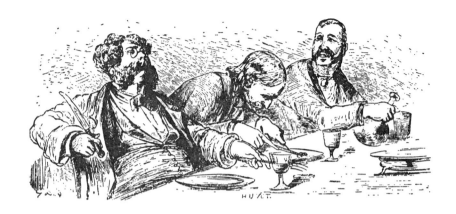

CUTTING CHOLESTEROL COMFORTABLY

When I had to cut down my cholesterol level, I overreacted and almost made a silly mistake in planning my diet. Here are some low-cholesterol diet tips I learned the hard way.

"Your cholesterol is up a bit," Dr. Kurzman told me. At my look of alarm, he held up his hand. "You're still in the normal range, but it's a high normal. See if you can get it down."

I left his office promising myself that now I would go on that diet I had thought about for so long. I was easily ten pounds overweight, and with a high normal cholesterol . . .

But ten pounds is so easy to hide, especially if you're tall, and after all I was still in the normal range. It wasn't that crucial or Dr. Kurzman would have been a lot tougher. So I let things drag on until my favorite pair of pants wouldn't close comfortably. That did it. I would start dieting that Monday!

"Why not today?" my wife asked.

"We have this dinner date on Saturday, and I hate to miss Sunday breakfast with the kids—and anyway, all good diets start on Monday."

That Sunday afternoon I was taking a walk in the country with my neighbor John, and we topped a small rise that looked down on a green field. John nodded at the orderly rows of plants. "Do you know that the answer to the future is in that field."

"What do you mean?"

"Soybeans. That field is planted with soybeans, and it's going to yield 450 pounds of protein for each acre."

"I still don't follow you."

He pulled a strand of grass and chewed its end. "Do you know how much it costs to raise animals for food? Or, to turn it around, how much animal protein you get per acre if you use the land to raise grain to feed animals? Forty-three pounds of protein! You get more than ten times that if you raise soybeans. I tell you, meat is on its way out. It's tomorrow's great luxury."

"It's today's luxury as well," I said, thinking of what I had paid for a steak the day before.

I kept thinking about John's comparison that night, and I began to dig through my books on nutrition. Was there really enough protein in vegetables to support a healthy diet? What effect would an all-vegetable diet have on the body's cholesterol?

I was surprised to find that cooked soybeans did very well—11 percent protein. This is about half of what you get in meat, fish, or cheese. If I included nuts, peas, and beans in my vegetable diet, I could get all the protein I needed. But I didn't intend to become a permanent vegetarian. I just wanted to stay on the diet until my weight was right and my cholesterol was down.

The more I read through the literature, the more convinced I became that we Americans all eat too much meat, perhaps too much protein. But eliminating meat would also eliminate the saturated fat in my diet. Logically, my body should respond by releasing its stored-up cholesterol.

"Monday is the first day of my cholesterol-free life," I told my wife.

"And how will you manage it?"

"With a vegetarian diet."

"What a strange coincidence!" she said brightly. "Monday I have a number of appointments—for lunch and dinner, to be exact. You'll be on your own."

I quickly realized that the problem was the very bad press that vegetarian food has been given. In my wife's eyes I was already wearing saffron robes and chanting "Hare Krishna." There had to be a better way, and a bright thought occurred to me. "But you do like Chinese food?"

"Love it."

"Well—there you are. I'm simply going on a Chinese food kick—for maybe thirty days."

"Without meat? I'd hate it."

I did some instant compromising. "Meat, no, but fish, yes, and chicken. Just think, chicken in hoisin sauce, sweet and sour sea bass, shrimp with black beans, crab and beancurd soup . . ."

"I'll try it—for a week." She thought for a moment. "But it's your diet. You do the cooking."

I broadened my research to include the art of Chinese cooking and with the help of Joyce Chen and Madame Chu, I worked out a careful set of menus for the first week. I wasn't prepared to plan for a whole month till I finished that first week. I dusted off the wok, polished the chopsticks, and we entered our Oriental phase.

I eliminated all butter, meat, and egg yolk from my diet, but I bought some safflower oil to cook with. It's as polyunsaturated as you can get. Pork and beef and lamb and all fat poultry became no-nos. I shopped for my chicken in Chinatown where there were none of those estrogen-fatted birds you pick up in the supermarket, and I bought only lean fish—no salmon, bluefish, sardines, herring, or shad.

Desserts were fresh fruit, and I used all the vegetables available. I used the high-protein pasta for my lo mein. The only problem was breakfast. I couldn't stick to the Chinese theme there, so I settled for fruit, cereal, and sugarless bread.

Wherever possible, I eliminated sugar. My reasoning there was from the gut. I had read so much about the harmful effects of sugar that I didn't think its loss would hurt me. At first I missed the candy, cake, and ice cream, but after a while, the act of sacrifice became its own reward. There's a bit of martyr in all of us.

I also cut out whole milk and whole-milk products—not so much for weight loss, but for cholesterol clearance. I drank skim milk for breakfast and eliminated coffee—again for no reason except that somewhere I had read that caffeine was linked to cholesterol.

The first week was intriguing. "You've got quite a touch with the wok," my wife admitted.

"Are you game for another week?"

"You do the cooking, and I'll eat along."

My pants fitted comfortably by the end of the first week, and at the end of the month I presented myself at Dr. Kurzman's office. "I want a retake on that cholesterol." I told him.

When the results came back, he sat down with me frowning thoughtfully. "That's very remarkable. Your physical health is fine, and I like the way you've lost weight, but your cholesterol level is what I'm amazed at. It's way down. You've become a low normal. Now, that's fine, but just what did you do?"

I told him about my Chinese diet and he nodded. "Of course. There's a group of investigators out in California—I think they call themselves the Longevity Institute—who claim to have reversed heart disease with a diet like yours. Of course, they cut out all fat. You used safflower oil."

"I had to use some oil with Chinese cooking."

"I don't think they bother with gourmet food. They work with far-gone patients, people in their late seventies and eighties. They cut out all smoking, fats, sugar, salt, all foods with cholesterol, and coffee and tea. And they claim some remarkable results. Cholesterol levels drop, and when they combine the diet with exercise, jogging, or walking, they say it cures angina, hypertension, and even diabetes. You ought to go whole hog and eliminate all the fat and see what happens."

"But I haven't got heart disease!"

"That's true." He looked at me speculatively. "Maybe I'll try it on some of my really bad patients. If it works, it's really the ultimate diet." He shuffled my reports. "Very remarkable. Invite me over for one of your Chinese dinners, and maybe I'll try the diet myself."

THE ULTIMATE DIET

For lunch, choose one from column A.

For dinner, choose two from column A, one from column B.

Breakfast is Occidental: juice, herb tea or decaffeinated coffee, matzo or dried toast from sourdough bread, cereal without sugar or butter. Artificial sweetener is fine, but artificial margarine is not.

Note: To cook these dishes in the wok, use the smallest possible amount of safflower oil. When you follow a recipe, quarter the oil and make up for it by stirring more rapidly. If the food is stirred constantly over moderate heat, it won't burn. You can substitute artificial sweetener for sugar in any recipe. All the dishes listed can be found in any good Chinese cookbook. The cutting, chopping, and careful preparation needed to cook Chinese style is an added pleasure.

COLUMN A	COLUMN B
Cabbage and dried shrimp soup	Chicken with green peppers
	Chicken in hoisin sauce
Fried rice	Chicken with walnuts
Hot and sour soup (Omit the pork)	Shrimp with black beans
	Steamed whole carp
Lo mein	Sweet and sour sea bass

COLUMN A

Braised eggplant, Szechuan
style (Omit pork)
Mushrooms with beancurd
Buddha's delight
Any vegetable in season,
stir-fried

COLUMN B

Red cooked fish
Poached fish, Canton style

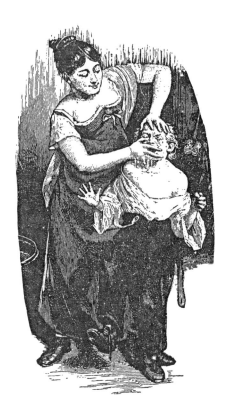

ABOUT
FACE

Treat your face right and you'll feel good all over.

"According to a recent article in a gossip column," Sandra tells a group of us over coffee at Marianne's apartment, "Paul Newman keeps his head in a bucket of water for twenty minutes every day!"

What can you say to a statement like that? "Without drowning?" I ask.

"He uses a snorkel, of course."

"Of course!" Raymond nods. "But what's the point?"

"His skin. It moisturizes his skin. If you're a movie actor, always under those lights, it's tremendously important to keep your skin moist."

"All I ask is to keep it free of acne," Bruce sighs. "My life didn't start until I hit twenty and my acne faded away."

"You have good skin," Marianne says thoughtfully, looking closely at Bruce. "But you could do with a facial."

"A facial? For me?" Bruce laughs. "Now, that's a new one! A facial for a man!"

"Hollywood actors have them regularly," Sandra says, "and you should listen to Marianne. She ran a beauty school in Paris, and she has a doctorate in chemistry."

Marianne waves that away. "The truth is, I studied with Dr. Nadine Payot for many years at her Paris clinic."

"Who was she?" I ask.

"A Russian woman who had to go to the University of Lausanne to get her M.D. She became intrigued with skin care and opened a clinic in Paris in 1925." Marianne sighs. "What an inspiration that woman was." She looks at Bruce thoughtfully. "You could really use a facial. Your problem is that you have too oily a skin."

"Is that what causes acne?" Bruce asks.

"It causes the acne to become worse, but acne itself is a result of a hormonal imbalance. You seem to be over it. It's just that oily skin like yours needs special care, or it can easily lead to pimples and blackheads."

"But a facial . . ."

Marianne, slim and elegant in her one-shoulder white jersey gown, stands up with sudden determination. "Right here and now I'm going to give you a facial. You just sit there." She glides out of the room while Bruce looks after her with an adoring puppydog smile. "Is she serious?"

"I think she is," Sandra smiles. "You don't know how lucky you are. Marianne charges a fortune for this kind of attention."

Marianne returns with towels and a case of cosmetics. "Now, sit there and lean back. That's right." She arranges Bruce on an overstuffed chair with a low back so he can rest his head comfortably. Then she drapes him with towels. "The first thing to remember," she tells us, "is that any facial must be effective, yet gentle enough not to rob the skin of its acid mantle."

"What is the acid mantle?" Raymond asks.

"The pH of the skin—the degree of acidity. The skin should be slightly on the acid side. That's nature's protection. Most soaps are alkaline, and they neutralize the skin. I prefer neutral or even slightly acid soaps. Their use will leave the skin slightly on the acid side.

"The first step is cleansing the skin." She takes the top off a flat jar and pats a light cream on Bruce's skin as he melts under her touch. "Close your eyes. This is a cleansing emulsion to take the dirt and excess sebum out of your pores. Blocked pores with dried-out sebum create blackheads. This cream is slightly acid and won't foam, but it cleans."

Marianne pats the emulsifier all over Bruce's face, over his eyelids and nose, cheeks and neck, and then, with cleansing tissues, she wipes his face slowly, showing us the dirty tissues. "You see what comes off an apparently clean skin."

She has a bowl of water with her and she lathers up a hard-milled soap and scrubs it into Bruce's face with a silk brush. "I use a rotating motion with the brush. It's too delicate to hurt the skin, but it cleanses it again.

"Now the mask." She reaches into her case and comes out with a big tube. She squeezes a few inches of a heavy green cream onto her hand and begins to pat it all over Bruce's face, leaving only his eyes and lips free. In a few minutes he has the look of a wild mime. "This is a mint astringent mask," she tells us. "It shrinks the clean pores, and it picks up any dead skin or stale skin products."

"Like a mud pack?" Bruce asks.

"Exactly. Some people use mud, and some even use plaster of paris. The heat that setting plaster generates is very healthy for the skin."

"And it's not dangerous?" Raymond asks.

Marianne laughs. "Haven't you ever made a life mask? Of course it's not dangerous. But my mint mask is easier to handle, and I believe it's better. How do you feel now, Bruce?"

"This is a great trip. I think this stuff is far out. Keep patting me, and I'll float."

"We'll take your mask off now," Marianne says firmly. "I think it's been on long enough." She scrapes the mask away from some spots and lifts it from others. Under the mask Bruce's skin is firm and rosy.

"Now the moisturizing cream," Marianne says. "But I'll use an antiseptic drying lotion first, just to tone up the skin. I'm really going to massage the moisturizing cream in. I want you to close your eyes and relax completely."

"And stop whimpering!" Raymond laughs as Marianne starts her facial massage.

"That's ecstasy!" Bruce moans.

"There are certain things you must remember when you treat oily skin," Marianne says in a businesslike way. "The oil must be let out. You can't stop it in, or the pores will plug up. In fact, that's what acne is: plugged and infected pores. If Bruce really wants a fine skin, he should use a mask at least two times a week—maybe more. The mask keeps the oil flowing through his pores, and it also tightens up the pores.

"Close your jaws while I massage the cheek muscles. Now open your mouth. Good. See, I massage not the cheekbones but the soft tissue."

As she talks, Marianne massages Bruce's cheeks and runs her fingers down the lines at the corners of his mouth. With her middle fingers she massages his nose, every once in a while adding a bit more moisturizing cream. She does around the eyes, between the eyebrows and along the upper ridge of the cheekbones.

"I do this for at least five minutes. Do you like it?"

Bruce softly moans, "Don't stop!"

"Silly!" But Marianne is pleased. "Now the forehead and temples, from the center to the corner of the eyes. I do the neck with my palms, and the neck is important. It gives the clue to tension. Now the front of the neck to avoid a double chin."

"But I'm not even thirty!" Bruce protests. "How can I have a double chin?"

Marianne reaches down and pats his stomach. "You may not be thirty, but your body is long past it. You haven't taken good care of yourself. You need some exercise."

"I need a reason. I'll exercise for you, Marianne."

Laughing, Marianne soaks a small towel in hot water at the sink inside and one in cold. When she comes back she places the hot towel over Bruce's face, leaving an opening for his nose. "You do this very gently, never pressing the hot towel down. We just want moist heat. Now the cold towel to close the pores and firm up the skin. How do you feel?"

"Sensational." He touches his face, smiling blandly. "It feels like a baby's ass." He takes Marianne's hand. "Let's not waste it. Let me take you out tonight."

We all laugh and Marianne says, "You should keep that up now. Remember: at least twice a week."

"But I've got dry skin," Sandra says. "What do I do?"

"The same thing," Marianne says, "but concentrate on giving your skin extra lubrication. Make sure the creams you use are all moisturizing. Avoid astringents and use a penetrating cream under your makeup—something with shark liver oil. That's a lot like the natural oils your skin lacks."

"I'm a Capricorn," Sandra sighs. "Capricorns always have skin trouble."

"Nonsense," Marianne says firmly. "It's not in your stars, it's in your genes. Forget about astrology and look for moisturizers."

Still stroking his face, Bruce says, "What about tonight?"

"We'll discuss that later. Now let's have some coffee."

People of both sexes are discovering the secret once known by only a select group of women—the relaxation value of an expert facial. Give your husband or wife—or lover—a gift certificate to a professional facial salon for Valentine's Day. A touch of hedonism is always appreciated.

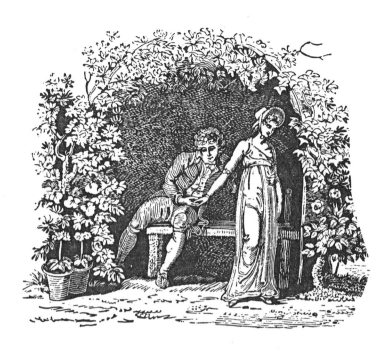

THE SECRET
OF THE AGES

The first encounter with sex is a learning experience, one of the most important ones of a person's life. Here's how one man learned something more meaningful than the technique alone.

Over some late brandy we had been talking about how well we remembered our early sexual experiences. Thoughtfully, Alan said, "I can remember the most tender, sensitive sexual experience—and the most horrifying!"

"I suppose it's natural to remember the two extremes," Claude said "I can recall some horrifying experiences of my own—but tender and sensitive? Let me see ..."

Alan laughed. "I can't forget because it was the same experience, the same woman."

"Tender, sensitive, and horrifying?" I asked. "You'll have to explain that."

Leaning back with a smile, Alan nodded. In his fifties, he was still a handsome man, broad-shouldered and over six feet tall, his blond hair streaked with gray but his bright blue eyes as youthful as ever. I could look at him now and see the young man he must have been.

"I was eighteen," he said slowly, "and still a virgin. You've got to remember that this was before the so-called sexual revolution. Most of us were still virgins at that age, and most of us denied it staunchly. We discussed sex very knowingly and boasted—reluctantly, understand—about our sexual conquests.

"It was the summer of 1940, and I had my first paying job as a waiter at a boy's camp. It was a great job. I worked during meals, and for a few minutes before and after, and had the time of my life. There was a little hotel attached to the camp, mainly to take care of the few visiting parents, and we waiters could often earn a few extra bucks by doing odd jobs for the guests.

"My best friend Dan was a waiter too—in fact he had gotten me the job—and his mother was one of the more permanent guests. She had another younger son who was a camper, and she spent most of the summer at the hotel. There was no husband around, and from what my friend said, I guessed that his parents had been separated for years—and he was still bitter about it.

"Elsie, his mother, was one of the best tippers in the hotel, and one of the pleasantest women. She was very small, hardly up to my shoulders, and very slim. That alone was unusual in those days. All mothers, almost by definition, were like mine, heavy and motherly. Elsie was the least motherly woman I knew, and one of the most helpless. She was always calling the front office for help with this or that—and the front office took the easy way out by sending over a waiter. For some reason, I was always the waiter.

"Elsie would smile with relief when I showed up and she'd explain the problem with an implied 'Thank goodness it's you.

No one else could open this stuck window, fix the hole in this screen, change the light bulb, move this trunk or whatever.' "

Alan shook his head. "And I'd be clumping around, a big lummox in shorts and sneakers, eager to please her because you just couldn't help wanting to please Elsie, and then—Christ, I don't know how or just when it happened. It seemed that she was a little more grateful each time, and a little more friendly and she would touch my arm or sometimes my chest if I was without a shirt—and anyway, one day I just had her in my arms and I was damned if I knew how it happened.

"She was very gentle and I was terrified. I blurted out my innocence and she just smiled and drew me down on the bed and—what can I say? It was the most tender, sensitive sexual experience I have ever had since. And it didn't stop there. It went on all summer. I'd sneak over whenever I could, day or night and she never rejected me or put me off. She was always willing, patient, eager, and so understanding. I can only say, after all these years, thank God for older women. Elsie conditioned me sexually to think of all women as warm, gentle, and sensitive."

There was a long pause, and I could sense Alan's mind turning back in time toward that summer. "But you called it horrifying," I said finally. "I don't understand."

"Don't you?" He looked at me over the rim of his brandy glass. "She was my best friend's mother. Dan and I worked together, shared the same tent, and went to town on dates together—and I was taking his mother to bed at least once a day! That was horrifying. I never spoke to Dan again after that summer, and he never knew why. You've no idea of the mixture of relief and despair that filled me when that summer was over and I said good-bye to Elsie."

"And guilt?"

"Hell, guilt had been with me all along."

Claude laughed. "But the real point of your story that strikes home is the pleasure a young man can get from an older woman. When I was that age I had just started the university in Paris, and I was introduced by a friend to an older woman, a nurse." He was silent for a moment, chewing his lip. Then he shook his head. "I too was an innocent, and she was"—he shrugged—"twenty years older than I. Good-looking, but perhaps with a touch of despair that her youth was gone. I don't know. How do you analyze these things in retrospect? I can only remember the pleasure of the years I spent with her, my years at the university. My fellow students were—what do they call it now?—all strung out and filled with sexual tension. I had none of that. I saw Nanette each morning on my way to school. She'd have just come off night duty, and I'd drop into her rooms. She'd cook her dinner and my breakfast and we'd go to bed, and than I'd leave her for classes and she'd sleep. We had only that involvement—only those morning hours—but it was enough for both of us."

"You didn't want a social life, either of you?" I asked curiously.

"No. You see, her friends were too old and mine too young. It was perfect as it was." He sighed. "I don't know whether I learned more in classes or in my nurse's bed, but looking back now, I can honestly say it was the most pleasant sexual experience of my life. Not the most passionate or the most exciting, but certainly the most pleasant. I give you a toast to older women." He lifted his glass.

I lifted mine, suddenly remembering a warm and accommodating librarian I had known when I too was a teen-ager. How long ago it was, and I had all but forgotten. But now, in a rush of pleasure, it all came back. Of all the love affairs in my life it was certainly the least complicated and one of the pleasantest, and my librarian had been how old? Forty, when I was in my late teens!

Smiling, I said, "I'll drink to that!"

If you're a woman, an older man might be able to give you the same sensitivity and maturity that these older women gave their younger partners. In a later chapter, I'll tell you what some younger women said about sex with older men.

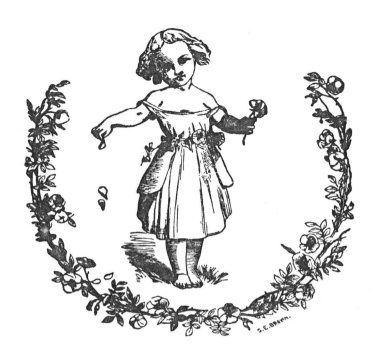

LOOK GOOD, FEEL GOOD

If you know how to use the right cosmetics, looking good can mean feeling good, too.

I met Gloria on the long ridge up behind my house. She was wearing jeans and a loose gauze overblouse, her long brown hair tumbling down her back, her green eyes glowing. She had a paper bag with her and was carefully filling it with wild rose petals.

I said, "Hi, neighbor." Then, curiously, "I can see picking flowers, but picking petals?"

"For an *enfleurage*," she told me and at my blank look went on to explain. "It's the way I get the scent out of the petals. Here, smell them."

I sniffed at the bag, half-full of petals. "Lovely! Can you really get that same scent?"

"Oh, yes. I use large, clear glass jars, and I put a layer of cotton in the bottom, then an inch or so of rose petals, then wet it down with some kind of bland, unscented oil—safflower or peanut. Then another layer of cotton, petals, and oil until the jar is full."

"Then what?" I asked fascinated.

"Oh, then I let the jar stand in the sun, or some nice warm place for a day or two, and then I press out the oil from the cotton and I have my attar of roses, my *enfleurage*."

I helped Gloria fill her paper bag with petals. "I have to pick them at dusk or sunrise when the flowers are moist and dewy, not dried out," she said.

Afterward we cut through the woods to her place, a small house she has built almost single-handedly. "Have a cup of tea and you can watch me start the *enfleurage*," Gloria suggested. I accepted a hot glass of herb tea—dried elephant ears carefully steeped and flavored with wild honey—while I watched her prepare her rose-petal mixture.

"What do you use the oil of roses for?" I asked, and Gloria looked up at me with wide, startled eyes.

"Why, for cosmetics, of course."

I was bewildered on two counts. First, I never knew that Gloria used cosmetics. She's an ardent advocate of the natural life in every aspect. Second, the idea of making cosmetics seemed too complicated to me. She would surely need a laboratory. "Do you really use cosmetics?" I asked.

She laughed at that. "Just like a man. Don't tell me you never noticed."

"And I thought that peaches-and-cream complexion was natural!"

"That peaches-and-cream complexion comes from just that—peaches and cream. For heaven's sake, don't look so betrayed. Women have been using cosmetics ever since Eve smeared hibiscus juice on her cheeks to make them redder and found that it closed the pores up very nicely."

I sip at my tea, shaking my head. "Poor Eve!"

"Poor Adam! Oh, I know. You're wondering how it all fits in with my attitude toward natural things, but that's just it. I won't use store-bought cosmetics with all their phony additives and artificial stabilizers. I make my own out of what's available plus a few natural ingredients I buy at the drugstore."

"Tell me about some of them."

"Well . . ." She considers for a moment, then jumps up and goes to her bathroom, returning with a mason jar of pale yellow lotion. "Take this. You mentioned peaches and cream, and this is made of both."

"But how?"

"I take two tablespoons of light cream and add the same amount of peach juice without sugar. Then I stir in a quarter of a cup of very strong tea. When it's smooth, I add three tablespoons of witch hazel, very slowly, stirring till it's smooth, and there it is,—a terrific facial cooler. Try some."

I rub a bit on my face and I'm surprised at the coolness and the refreshing quality of it. "Wonderful! What else do you make?"

"I make just about everything I need, but let's take the basic cosmetic every woman uses."

"Lipstick?"

"Don't be silly. Cold cream, and I use a really old-fashioned recipe. I get my beeswax from the same place I get my wild honey."

"From bees?"

"From a friend's hive. I boil the wax to get rid of the impurities, and I melt about half a cup of it with half a cup of very pure olive oil. I do it in a double boiler and blend them well. Then I add half a cup of heavy mineral oil, the kind you get in any drugstore."

"And that's cold cream?"

"Not yet. I dissolve a teaspoon of borax in five ounces of water, bring it to a simmer, and slowly add the wax mixture, beating it all the time. I take it off the heat and beat it till it's smooth, then add a few drops of my rose scent and put it in a nice clean jar. It thickens as it stands and becomes a great cold cream base."

"What other cosmetics do you make?"

Gloria digs into a can and comes up with some granola cookies. "Try these. Let's see, you asked about lipstick. I don't use it, but sometimes I use a lip gloss. I make that with beeswax, olive oil and mink oil."

"What on earth is mink oil?"

"Just what it seems. An oil rendered from the fat of the mink. It's very polyunsaturated, and it's super for the skin. Also, there's a great body lotion I make from egg yolks and honey."

"Who gets to lick it off?"

"I've been known to become edible afterward. It starts with a gel made from slippery elm, one part of the shredded bark to three parts of water. You cook it for half an hour and then strain it through a coffee filter and let it stand. It becomes a gel.

"Then you add four tablespoons of it to two egg yolks. And four tablespoons of honey, two tablespoons of sesame seed oil, and half a cup of fresh milk. It's a tremendous moisturizer for the skin,—soothing, too. And I usually stir in a bit of my flower scent, too.

"Oh, there's no end to the stuff you can make to perk up your skin and hair—and all of it with natural material. Some one wrote an entire book on it, and I use that for my basics. Then I wing it from there."

"You mean you make up your own cosmetics?"

"Oh yes. For instance, there's a great herbal mix for the face. You take a strong tea, about four times as strong as you would drink, and dilute it with one cup of water and one teaspoon of tapioca. Strain it through some filter paper and let it cool. You've got a soothing lotion for burns or inflammations, but the tea's the loose part."

"What do you mean?"

"Well, I can vary it. I can use regular tea, or any kind of herb tea, or even sassafras root."

"Sassafras root?"

"Sure. It's the flavor they use for birch beer. You boil the root to extract the essence. The tapioca makes it into a gel."

"You know, it sounds so interesting I'm sorry men don't use cosmetics."

"Are you kidding? Of course you do. What about after-shave lotion? You can make a great one by blending a whole lime with a cup of witch hazel, a half cup of ethyl alcohol, a teaspoon of corn syrup, and two egg whites. Filter the result, and have you got an after-shave lotion!"

"That I'm going to try," I promise, and I walk home through the evening dusk eagerly searching for flowers to begin depetaling tomorrow.

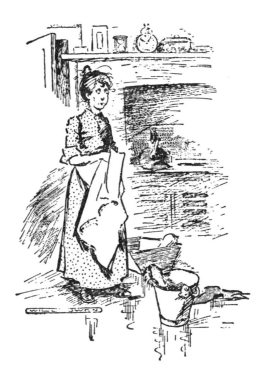

EXTRA EFFORT
THE EASY WAY

Working harder at your exercise program isn't the only way to get more out of it. You might try a different kind of extra effort.

The first time I noticed Jenny's perambulations was when she had me over for lunch. I hadn't seen her since the birth of her second baby, and I was delighted to find her full of vitality and fun. And best of all—she had lost all the extra weight she put on during pregnancy.

After the soup, Jenny cleared the table, but only one dish at a time. Then she began bringing in the salad, again one dish at a time. When she finally sat down, I said, "You know, you could use a time-and-motion man around this house."

Jenny laughed. "Haven't you caught on?"

"To what?"

"To the fact that I'm doing it all deliberately. I make four trips to do what I could in two, or even one. It's the same way when I clean up. I do it with the maximum amount of walking. I make a dozen trips to the kitchen and to my cleaning cupboard. I walk around the bed four times when I make it. In fact, I do just about everything with two or three times the effort I need."

"But I don't understand!" I said in genuine bewilderment. "If you know you're being so inefficient, why keep doing it?"

"Efficiency is a matter of definition. I'm being a very inefficient housewife, yes, but I'm being very efficient as an exerciser."

"Oho!" A light begins to dawn. "You do this all for exercise, to give yourself a workout?"

"Exactly. You might say I go all around the mulberry bush instead of stepping over it. But you see, I'm tied down to the house these days. I'm really and truly a housewife now. Oh, not that I fight it or resent it. The children are darling, and I love them, and I've set up the attic as a studio. I do get to paint during their naps—when I'm not having someone to lunch like now—I'll take you up there later."

"But you've got to explain more about this—this all-around-the-mulberry-bush routine."

"It's very simple. Here, try some of this bread. I baked it myself."

"With how many trips to the oven and back?"

"That's it exactly. You put your finger on it. I've done away with shortcuts and efficiency around the kitchen and the house—and I've done it very deliberately. Here I am, trapped in this house all day with the children. I used to be a very active woman, but I've had to give up tennis and skiing—all the things Tom and I did before the babies."

"And you want to keep from getting fat?"

"Oh, no—or oh, yes. I do want to keep from putting on all the housewifely flab, but that's diet. I watch what I eat and I stay thin. The exercise is something else. I do it to keep in shape, to keep my body toned up, my muscles working."

"And just what do you do?"

"Well, basically, whenever I can, I move. That's the key to it. I double and triple the number of trips I make around the house. I sit down and get up a dozen times during a meal. When I'm tending the baby or cleaning I bend and stretch and go about it in the most vigorous way I can. And getting things. I never ask Tom to get me something from the next room. I get up and get it myself. He thinks I'm a devoted wife, but the truth is I'm selfish. If I were all that devoted, I'd let him move his butt a bit; as it is, I do it all for that extra movement I get out of it."

Amused, I asked her, "Is all this inefficiency something you indulge in only around the house?"

"Oh, no. Outside, too. When I take a bus home, for instance, I get off two or three stops before my regular one, and I walk the difference—if I take a bus at all. Any distance under two miles I walk!"

"You must save a lot of money in carfare."

"Right, but what's more to the point is what I spend, I mean in energy. I look on all these little tricks, the extra walking, the stairs—do you know, I can't remember when I last took an elevator or an escalator in a shopping center. I walk up and down every flight of steps I can find. Well, all of this—I look on them all as something I'm putting over on everyone else."

"I don't quite get that."

"What I mean is, I don't consider any of this a task, something I must do. I never get annoyed at jumping up from the table to fetch things. I don't grumble when I run up and down the stairs to take care of the babies. It's not something I have to do, but something I want to do. I don't complain to myself about all the extra work."

"How can you help it?"

"Simply by looking at it all as a sort of game. You see, I'm the one who's gaining by all this. I'm not being taken advantage of. It's turning things around like that that makes it all fun—or at least as much fun as real honest-to-goodness exercise."

"Which isn't always fun."

"Well, of course it isn't and this isn't always fun either. Especially when I'm tired—but neither is it self-sacrifice or hard work. It's exercise, with all the pluses and minuses of exercise. It's exercise I want to do, and as long as I look at it from that viewpoint, it isn't a drag."

Jenny reaches across the table for another slice of bread. "And of course it does burn up some extra calories,—enough to indulge in an extra nibble here and there. Have some more of this. Isn't it good?"

"It is. I'll have some more if I can take my dishes into the kitchen and bring back a cup of coffee—myself!"

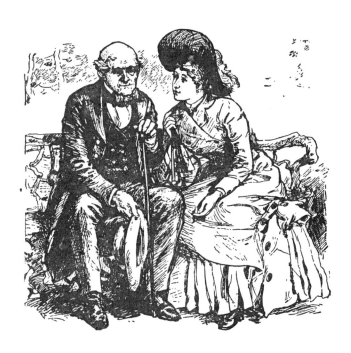

THE SECRET
OF THE AGES—
ANOTHER VIEW

Younger women in search of romance and fun sometimes aren't satisfied with what they find—perhaps because they've been operating under the wrong assumption. Here's another approach to try.

"You can praise older women all you want," twenty two-year-old Mary Ann told me firmly. "For myself, I'll take an older man any time."

I looked across the dance floor in the small supper club where Mary Ann's "date" Richard was dancing with my wife. Richard was in his early fifties, slim and erect. He still had all his hair cut short in a pepper-and-salt crew cut, and a handsome, craggy face. He was also an extremely successful businessman.

"Richard has a lot going for him," I admitted. "I like him, and I'll admit he's fun to be with, but—"

"But me no buts!" Mary Ann said firmly. "We're not getting married. It's just an affair and we both know it—but it's one hell of a great affair!"

"Even with some thirty years' difference in age?"

"Even so."

"Well, tell me about it."

Mary Ann smiled and brushed her long blond hair back from her face. "I met Richard on an airplane. We were both coming into Chicago from New York, and we had a long talk— a very pleasant talk—and he bought me a couple of drinks. Then he offered me a lift home. He was parked at the airport, and I accepted. I had started off thinking of him as—well, a fatherly type. He was certainly old enough to be my father, but somewhere along the ride home the father figure disappeared."

I must have looked dubious because she frowned a bit. "Yes, I know it's popular psychology to think that a young girl and an older man is simply a case of the girl's looking for daddy, but it wasn't that way with me. For one thing, I have a perfectly good daddy of my own, not too possessive and— well, anyway, I asked Richard up for a drink and one thing led to another—not to bed that first night, though I think he could have coaxed me into it if he wanted to, but he was too considerate—and that's the key to the whole thing."

"Being considerate?"

"In a way—or perhaps being mature. When I've had other men up to my apartment, men closer to my own age, and it became obvious that we liked each other, they'd push for as much as they could get. I think it's a male macho thing. Most men are terrified of being thought unmanly, and to them manly means going as far as they can."

"Isn't that a little—well, too harsh on them?"

"Is it? All I can say is it always happens. Richard is the first older man I've gone with, and it didn't happen. There was no doubt in my mind that he wanted sex, and I did, too, but he moved slowly." She smiled over my shoulder and I turned to watch Richard and my wife come back to the table.

I saw Mary Ann for lunch a week later, and I asked, "How is the Affair Richard?"

"You can laugh, but I'm in love."

"Then it has matured?"

"We've slept together, and it's been all I expected. What more can I say?"

"I think I envy Richard, or do I? I don't think, at his age, I could keep up an affair with a young girl. I'd be too tired. How could I explain taking a nap every night during the news program?"

Mary Ann laughed. "I'm the one who naps before dinner. The point is, an affair doesn't have to be a swinging young thing. We don't go at my pace, and yet I don't think it's Richard's pace either. Sex with Richard is different. There's none of the wildness of young men, but there's more satisfaction." She pushed the salt cellar around the table, avoiding my eyes. "I've never understood the richness of sex before, how satisfying it can be. Oh, I enjoyed it, of course, but it was a fifty-fifty thing, I mean with men in my crowd, in my age group. Sometimes I'd have an orgasm, sometimes I wouldn't. With Richard I always do. Do you know what that means to a woman?"

"I think so, but why? Is it because of the way you feel about him, what you called being considerate when I first met him?"

"Considerate? Yes, that and maybe just his age. He's slower, and everything is more leisurely. I'm more relaxed, more together, I guess. There isn't the same intensity there is with young men, but there's a tranquillity that I love—and I'm learning."

"About sex?"

"Oh, about that, sure. I'm learning how men react, what they like and what they can do, and I'm learning it without pressure. But it's more than that. Richard knows more than I do. He's been to more places, seen more of life and done more. He's been married—you know, he's a widower, and he has grown children, and it's like every time we're together I find out a little more."

"About what?"

She shrugged. "Little things. How to order in a restaurant. What wines are good. We'll go to a museum and without pressure he'll open my eyes to color and form—and music! I've always liked classical stuff, but he's shown me the fine points, why I like it and what to look for. The theater too—even movies and TV. I guess so much of it is age. He smooths off my corners and my burrs, and he does it very gently, very lovingly."

"You *have* got a case!"

"Haven't I? I asked him to marry me the other night."

"What did he say?"

"The sensible thing. That he loved me very deeply, but we didn't really belong together permanently, and he was sure I'd realize it." She shook her head. "He said it was a matter of available time, he didn't have enough left and I had too much ahead of me. It was kind of sad and I wanted to cry, but he said I was silly. What we have now is wonderful, and we'd both treasure it years from now."

"It sounds like a soap opera."

"Doesn't it? I loved it. Oh, it didn't sound like that when he said it. It was very sweet and—you know, I think I felt relieved inside, because I know he's right. But it was a nice way to tell me."

"Even though you love him?"

"There's love and love. Richard says every time we love we grow a little. Maybe this is a period of growth for me."

I ordered coffee and shook my head. "I can see where it's going to be a lot of *Richard says* from now on!"

I didn't see Mary Ann for a number of months after that, and then one afternoon I ran into Richard at a midtown bar. We remembered each other, shook hands, and ordered drinks. "And how's Mary Ann?" I asked.

He smiled and reached back for his wallet. "She sent me this last week." He handed me a picture of two laughing young people in swimsuits. One was Mary Ann; the other was a good-looking young man. "They're engaged."

"Oh." I handed the picture back. "Do I say 'How nice' or 'I'm sorry'?"

" 'How nice,' of course. He's a fine youngster with good prospects, and I'm sure he'll make her very happy. I've met him."

I looked at him curiously. "You know, I've talked with Mary Ann about you."

He nodded. "Yes, she told me."

"And how do you feel about it all?"

He looked genuinely surprised. "Why, how should I feel? Pleased, of course. I loved her—still do—and we had a wonderful time together. Our age difference made marriage impossible—for me at least—and I don't think Mary Ann loved me that way. But this is the real thing, and good for her. I'm very happy."

I raised my glass. "I'm glad it's ended well. I'll drink to you both."

He smiled and lifted his glass, then looked past me and stood up abruptly. "Ah, here's my date. Let me introduce you."

I turned as a pretty, dark-haired young girl—in her twenties, at least—hurried toward us, her eyes on Richard, her smile like a candle in the dim bar. I sighed and took a deep drink. "To all young girls and older men," I whispered to myself.

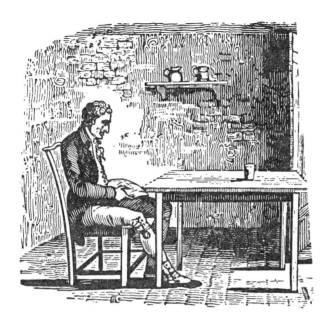

FAST
AND LOSE

*One of my friends believes that fasting can be a sensual high.
Here's her technique.*

I honestly believe that there is a higher spiritual plane,"
Regina tells me.

"Are you talking about life after death?" I ask. We have
been out for a walk in the late autumn, and there is a sharp
bite to the air. The trees—skeletons now, with only a few
tattered leaves clinging to them—look like Chinese brush-
strokes against a darkening sky.

We rest on a little hill that overlooks the cold waters of a
pond, and Regina pulls her heavy Mexican sweater around her
thin body. "No—although it may be related. I'm talking about
a plane of existence we can reach in this life, a state where you

become tremendously aware of everything physical as well as psychic."

I sit down on a low stone wall and say, "Back up now and explain that."

Her deep green eyes intense, Regina throws out her arms as if to embrace the sere landscape. "In the state I'm talking about, you could look at those trees and they'd glow with an aura of their own. Those hills wouldn't be that dingy mud color. They'd be an intense ultraviolet, and they'd have an aura above them—every living thing would have an aura!"

"You make it sound like a Peter Max illustration."

"Don't you think he had a vision of that place?"

"In my youth it was Maxfield Parrish who had the vision."

"Of course. The Beatles saw it, too—and I've seen it!"

"You have?" I'm genuinely surprised. "How did you do that?"

Regina drops down beside me on the wall. "By fasting."

Now I'm a bit shocked. Regina is such a wraith of a girl that it seems as if a heavy wind could blow her away. In fact, in some ways she seems a creature made of wind. "But surely you don't need to fast. You don't need to lose weight."

"Not now I don't, but then I did."

"When was then?"

"Let me see . . . it was over five years ago, and I had just graduated high school. Our yearbook printed our pictures with little one-liners. Mine was rather lethal. It read, 'A sideshow contender.' "

"What did that mean?"

"That I was headed for fat lady in a circus."

"How cruel!" I look at her again. "And how impossible."

"I weighed 200 pounds—on the nose."

"I don't believe it. You can't be more than 120 now."

Regina shrugs. "I don't know. I never weigh myself now. I just don't have a weight problem anymore. You see, my weight has stayed the way it is for five years. I know that because my clothes fit, and I don't bother with scales."

"Two hundred pounds! Where did you put it all?"

"All over, evenly. I really was a candidate for a circus fat lady, but that line under my picture shook me up. I decided I was going to lose it all, and right away. I decided to go on a real fast."

"For how long?"

Regina smiles. "You won't believe this, but I went without real food for three months."

"I find that hard to believe—but I find it even harder to believe that you were once fat."

Regina says, thoughtfully, "It's hard for me too. I don't think of myself as fat—but then, I never did. Maybe that was why I never tried to diet until—well, until my face was rubbed in it."

"Were you thin as a child?"

"Oh, yes, but it all changed when I hit adolescence."

"And it was fasting that made you aware of a higher spiritual plane?"

"How can I explain that without sounding like a kook?" Regina bit her lip. "It must have been about the fourth day of the fast. I was living in Cleveland then, and you know—it was all legitimate."

"How do you mean, legitimate?"

"Well, it wasn't just some way-out idea I got myself. Our family doctor suggested it when I told him I wanted to lose weight. I had the beginning of a problem with diabetes then— only, it cleared up with the weight loss. He wanted me to take it off fast, too, so he sent me to Mount Sinai Hospital where they were using what they called a protein-sparing fast. You have to be *real* careful with fasting."

"I know. For some people it can be very dangerous—deadly, in fact."

Regina nods, picking a dried branch from the ground and pulling off the leaves as she talks. "You should be thoroughly examined first, and I was. I spent the first week in the hospital, and afterward I saw my doctor once a week. It was during that first week that I had that altered perception, a sort of expanded awareness. I began to see auras around things, and I almost sensed the presence of another continuum."

"In short, you were hallucinating."

Regina laughs, poking at the dead leaves with her stick. "I know that—and I knew it then, but sometimes hallucinations are truer than reality."

I considered that for a moment, but I couldn't find a sound rebuttal. "To get back to your fast, isn't there a big danger that you can lose body protein? I know that the body first uses up the sugar stored in the liver, and you need sugar to survive. Since you can't get any sugar from your stored body fats, you break down your muscle protein. Now, that could damage the heart as well as the other body muscles."

"Exactly! That's why at Mount Sinai they made me take a special supplement with lots and lots of water to avoid stones forming in my kidney and bladder. Isn't that far out? I'd drink about eight glasses a day. That was the hardest part, but I got into the habit and I still drink a lot of water. Anyway, the supplement had glucose in it—that's the sugar the body uses— and minerals and amino acids. The body uses amino acids to make proteins, so even though I was fasting, I was taking in protein and sugar."

"But is that truly a fast?"

"Oh, well . . ." Regina shrugs. "Why do we always have to label and define things. I took in only 300 or 400 calories a day. Maybe that kept me from taking off an extra half pound of fat a week. The point is, I took it off—a couple of pounds every day in the beginning, then at least a pound a day. The funny thing is, I just wasn't hungry after the first three or four days."

"You found that higher spiritual plane."

"No—seriously, when I started, I thought I could never face up to a real fast; I needed food too much. But I surprised myself. You know, we used to have group sessions at the hospital while I was in the program, and my group decided that I had a thin self-image. I think maybe that's why I've kept it off."

"Do you recommend fasting to take off weight?"

"Not for everyone," Regina says quickly. "Some people can't—and shouldn't—and I'm a firm believer in fasting under a doctor's care. When I made reentry . . ."

"Reentry?"

"That's what we called beginning to eat again. I started with just one meal a day—all soft foods—and then I built up to the amount of food I needed for a stable weight. I've stayed with it ever since."

We stand up and start to walk back, the sharp wind whipping the leaves around us. "You know," Regina says thoughtfully, "you can combine fasting with your regular routine and fast only on weekends. You wouldn't need any special supplement or medical care."

"I'd hate that. We have our best meals on weekends."

"Or you could take two days during the week. That would take off weight, too. But the real answer, I think, is changing your whole life-style, your awareness of life."

"Is that what you mean by a higher plane of consciousness?"

"You've got it!" Regina gestures at the autumn woods, now almost in twilight. "Before my fast, I could never see things as sharply as I do now. Maybe my eyes are thinner, but I think—I really think it was that period of awareness that stayed with me."

"It wasn't just too many metabolized ketones in the brain?"

"No—or it wouldn't still be with me. And if it were just losing all that fat, well—it wouldn't have come to me so early in the fast. No, I really think I've gotten a glimpse of a higher spiritual plane."

"Well, let's get back to the house and have a hot drink or two and maybe I can sense it too," I tell her as we hurry home.

Before you try to lose weight by denying yourself food, get your doctor's permission. Over an extended period, fasting can endanger your health by depriving your body of essential nutrients and other important substances. According to medical authorities, fasting can be especially dangerous for anyone with a chronic disease such as diabetes.

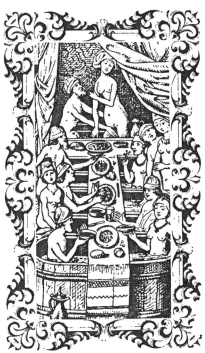

THAT CHAMPAGNE TOUCH

A few minutes of "treatment" with this technique can make anyone feel like a new person.

"Imagine a million delicate fingers probing your body gently, so gently they're almost a suggestion of a touch, and behind them a steady pressure—and all in a delicious heat in a most exquisite setting. How about that?"

"You're making my mind water," I tell Fred. "What and where and how?"

"The most sensual experience I've had in years. I was out in San Diego in California on a job interview, and some friends took me home to dinner. Afterward they said, 'How about a whirlpool bath in the back yard?'

"I couldn't believe them. They weren't kidding. Out behind the house they had a huge redwood deck, and in the center there was an enormous round tub, sort of like half a barrel, built out of wood. It must have been six feet across, and it was filled with bubbling water. It would have seated six of us comfortably, but we were only three—my host, his wife, and I. We shed our clothes and climbed in mother-naked, and what an experience!"

"Tell me."

"Well, the water must have been about 104 degrees, just hot enough to be pleasant without enervating you. They had some sort of whirlpool system under the porch, and streams of bubbling water shot into the tub from jets positioned below and on the sides. The water was foaming, and the bubbles would break against your skin like an effervescent drink. My host called it 'the champagne touch,' and he was right.

"There was a feeling of total luxury in those bubbles," Fred went on dreamily. Somehow they took the strength away from the jets of water but left a tingling touch. You were massaged constantly as you sat there, but so comfortably, so gently!

"There was a big redwood and glass screen set up in a semicircle around the tub to cut the wind, but it still let us see out over the garden, and, not too far off, the Pacific. We sat there endlessly and watched the sunset over the water, while the lovely Japanese garden behind us became dark and shapeless. It was a mind-blowing experience!

"Their whole house is built around that deck and tub. The entrance to the main house is through a bathroom behind the tub so that you can shower and dry off and get dressed— though you don't really have to shower. They chlorinate the tub water."

"I thought there were water shortages in California."

"Oh, well, yes—there sometimes are, but you see, those whirlpools are for health, and they're exempt from water rationing."

"Is that fair?"

"I think so. They really are healthy. If they don't help your physical health, they help your mental health. You spend an hour in one of those tubs, and you come out completely centered. It's a fabulous experience for your mental health— sort of a psychiatric tool."

"Ah—come on!"

"Seriously. Those tubs are better than liquor or grass. They calm you down amazingly, and the strange thing is, the calming process lasts."

"How long?"

"Oh, for hours afterward, and then you sleep like a baby. It's the greatest answer to insomnia I've ever seen."

"I've heard that about hot baths in general."

"Well, these whirlpool tubs are a step beyond baths. What's more, they're exciting—erotically exciting. A lot of people out there use the baths for sex."

"Now, that's a new one! How does sex enter in?"

"You have sex in the tub. It's very exciting. The hot water has erotic overtones, and the bubbles excite you—maybe because everyone bathes in the nude."

"Always?"

"Well, my friends do anyway. I visited a number of people out there, and almost all of them had the heated outdoor baths with the whirlpool attachments. With many of them, the tubs have replaced the swimming pool as a status symbol; but a lot of people have both, and that's a sensory high."

"In what way?"

"I was down in Santa Barbara on a chilly day—it was about 65 degrees, but the outside temperature didn't bother us because we were all up to our necks in our host's plastic whirlpool tub bath."

"Plastic?"

"This one was a bright red plastic. It looked great, and no matter how cold it was outside, the whirlpool was heated. That made all the difference in the world. What we'd do was run from the whirlpool tub to the swimming pool, and that was heated, too—but only to 75 degrees, and by contrast with the tub, it seemed cold. We'd plunge in and swim, and we'd get that contrast—hot and cold—but it was only a sensory contrast."

"What do you mean?"

"It was as if you jumped from the swimming pool into a very cold ocean. It was that sort of sensory shock, but that would be dangerous because the water is too cold. When you go from 104 degrees to 75 degrees you have the illusion of the same sort of shock, but it's not really cold, so there's no danger involved. Do you understand?"

"I think so."

"I really got into tub bathing when I was out there. It was just tremendous, a whole new sensory dimension in bathing. Now I'm checking out whirlpools for my bathtub at home. If I can find the right kind, I might install one."

"Would it be the same thing?"

"No, not really," Fred admits slowly. "The whirlpool—that champagne touch—is a good part of the whole thing, and I'm sure I could buy the equipment to duplicate it, but the ambience is almost as big a part. To me, tub bathing is all tied up with that beautiful wooden or plastic tub outside the house, the trees and shrubs, and, most wonderful of all, those incredible Pacific sunsets. You have no idea of the exquisite peace that floods through you as you sit there—and it's a social thing, too. You do it together with your friends and lovers."

I say thoughtfully, "You know, here in New York a lot of the old apartment houses have huge wooden tubs on their rooftops. If you could heat up one of those, you'd have the same thing as your back-yard tub. You could sit up there and watch the sun set over Jersey . . ."

"Very funny! But you're not all that far out. Tomorrow I'm visiting a friend with a penthouse, and he's talking about putting a wooden bathing tub out on his terrace. Man, I would really dig that. Imagine the champagne touch above New York City!"

"It boggles my mind!"

"I'll call you up when he gets it going."

Whirlpool baths have long been used in gyms and health spas by athletes who needed to relax tired muscles. Now they are becoming popular in resorts and in private homes—for anyone who wants to watch his pressures bubble away.

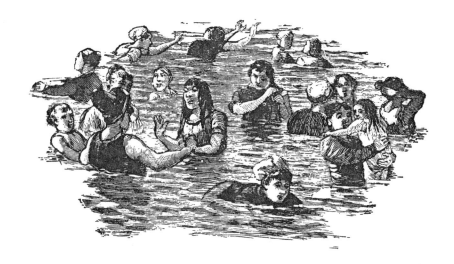

THE EASY ANSWER TO CROWDED POOLS

Swimming is said to be an ideal form of exercise, but what if the pool is so packed you can hardly dog-paddle three feet? That's no problem at all, if you know about schwimmflugel.

It's one of those wonderful summer days, hot and lazy, and a group of us are at the municipal pool where we have salvaged one small corner. Looking glumly at the mob of teen-agers splashing wildly, Lorna sighs. "I'll never get my workout."

Shirley asks, "Why not?"

Lorna gestures at the crowded pool. "Wall-to-wall kids, that's why not. Can you see me doing laps through that crowd?"

Sam, Lorna's husband, has stretched out lazily on the pool's edge, and he lets one hand trail in the water. "Why work out?

If you just relax and close your eyes, all that noise, that yelling and screaming, sounds like a waterfall. I can lie here in the sun and pretend I'm in a mountain pool with water cascading down behind me."

I shut my eyes a moment, then shake my head. "No way does that sound like a waterfall! It's kids, plain and simple."

"But you can still work out," Shirley insists. She pulls herself up on the pool's rim and reaches out for a round orange covered float with snaps on it. "I brought a few of these along."

"What are they?" Lorna inspects it curiously. "It's too small for water wings or a swim jacket—unless you snap two of them together."

"They're called swim floats," Shirley tells us. "I think they originated in Germany, where they call them *schwimmflugels*. They're made to snap on your wrists or ankles. Like this." She slips one on her wrist, where it looks like an enormous cuff or inflated bracelet. "See?"

Shaking my head, I say, "No. Are they to keep you afloat?"

"Well, they do, and that's the whole point. Here. Watch what happens when I put it on my ankle." She slips the flexible "cuff" off her wrist and over her foot to circle her ankle. "Now look." She slips down into the water and, predictably, her foot with the cuff attached rises to the surface. With a little frown of effort, Shirley pushes it underwater. "You have to work at keeping it down, you see, because you're working against gravity."

"Not really." I'm fascinated now. "You're working against the floating power of the cuff. It's as if you tried to pull down a helium-filled balloon."

"But I still don't see what that has to do with working out," Lorna says, puzzled.

"I have more of them," Shirley tells her. "Four, in fact. One for each wrist and ankle. They're over there by the lounge chair. Would you get them, Sam?"

With a grunt, Sam gets up and fetches the rest of the *schwimmflugels*. Clasping one on each wrist and the third on her ankle, Shirley floats on her back, a strange figure spread-eagled on the pool's surface. "Were they designed to keep you floating?" I ask curiously, squatting at the poolside.

"Yes, if you want to float like this," Shirley says. "But if you try to sit up, then you have to fight their floating power. See?" She pushes her two feet down and they promptly rise, spilling her onto her back. "I have to work to keep them down, and therein lies the secret!"

Lying flat on the water, she spreads her arms and legs, then brings her wrists and ankles together, her arms over her head. Then she brings her arms down to her side and spreads her legs. "That's a basic type of exercise, but you can see that it doesn't do much. You're all in one plane—the surface of the water—and you're not fighting anything."

A group of youngsters have come to watch, and one teenage boy asks, "What's the best exercise?"

Righting herself, Shirley says, "I think this one. You stand on tiptoes and kick out, raising your leg as high as you can, then pull it down. Then you do it with the next leg. I call it goose-stepping, and that's what it looks like. But you really feel it in your hips. Wow, do you feel it!"

"Why not just goose-step on land?" one of the girls asks.

"This is more fun, especially on a hot day, and it uses muscles you don't use on land. That's the fascinating thing about all these exercises. They work out a completely different set of muscles. When you're walking, you fight gravity—I guess." She looks at me and smiles. "But here you fight a different force, an upward force. Look." She snaps two of the floats on each leg, and with a frown of effort stands, then does a deep knee bend and straightens up. "Now that's work, real work."

"Let me try it," Lorna asks, and two of the teen-agers beg for a turn.

"I'll show you something you can do with just one," Shirley says, and snaps a float on each one's wrist. "You stand in water up to your shoulders, like this, and then lower your arm to your side. Then raise it and lower it. Let the float raise it, but you force it down."

"Oh, wow! That hurts," one of the young girls laughs, and

Lorna agrees. "I can feel my shoulders tensing and relaxing. You know, it has to be just the opposite of weight lifting."

"You can march, too," Shirley tells her fascinated audience. "You just put one float on each ankle and stand still and mark time in place, this time bending your knees. Or, if you're really strong, try two floats on each ankle."

"Let me!" a muscular teen-age boy begs, and Shirley snaps a double load on each of his legs. For a moment he stands, fighting the flotation power of the *schwimmflugels*. Then, with a yell, he flips backward, both his feet shooting up into the air. When Shirley finally gets him untangled, she demonstrates how it's done.

"It's a matter of balance, really, not pure muscle. What's great with a double ankle load is this one." She keeps two *schwimmflugels* on each ankle and reaches out to grab the poolside. "See? Holding the pool rim gives you the balance you need. Now you bring your knees up to your chest, then— oomph! Straighten them. Straight down. Feel what it does to your stomach muscles."

Most of the crowd of youngsters is around us now, and each one begs for a turn. Shirley shows them how to kneel and do a side kick, an arm circle, and a dozen other aquacalisthenics.

Watching in fascination, I finally turn to Sam and say, "You know, it looks like a wonderful exercise. It's not only good for the muscles—I can see that it stretches and pulls some you could never get to in the air, but it's also a novelty kind of thing. Look at the way the kids are eating it up."

"She's got the whole pool in this corner," Sam says, standing up with a grin.

"I'd like to try it myself."

"What? And miss an opportunity like this?" Sam gestures at the empty, waiting pool. "It's probably the only chance we'll get today to do laps. Come on!"

He dives in and streaks for the other side, and I follow him, the two of us with the pool to ourselves.

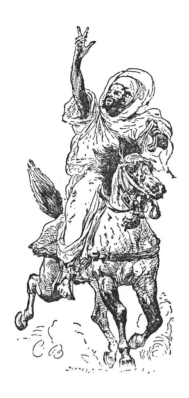

A GIFT FROM
GENGHIS KHAN

Maybe history has been unfair to Genghis Khan. He made one valuable contribution to my health and happiness—and he can do the same for you.

"Do you like the way my face looks?" I ask my wife.

"It looks the same as usual, except for your nose. That looks awful. Did you catch it in a door?"

"No. Actually, I had a fascinating experience with *Chua-ka*. I spent an hour having my face 'done,' and I must say I enjoyed it."

"Whoever did it was a bit rough on your nose."

"Let me tell you about *Chua-ka*. It was developed in the days of Genghis Khan to help take care of the battle wounds of his warriors."

"Who did this number on you?"

"He came well recommended. His name is Bob, and he trained at the Arica institute. I decided I'd try this instead of my usual massage. He explained that the principle of the massage is that not only the brain but the entire body remembers negative experiences and holds them. As long as these experiences are held, you tend to repeat them over and over—almost unconsciously."

"What has Genghis Khan got to do with that?"

"It seems that he realized that his warriors, once injured, would continue being injured again and again, and the more they tried to protect themselves, the more they'd be hurt. Do you get it?"

My wife looks at me curiously. "I get what you've said, but what does it mean—if anything?"

"These warriors of Genghis Khan discovered that they were their own worst enemies in the sense that the very act of trying to protect themselves hurt them, and the only way to stop the process was to purify their bodies with a very deep massage. That deep massage is *Chua-ka*."

"I wish you'd forget Genghis Khan and his warriors and tell me about the massage."

"It's based on the assumption that the body has different zones where different negative charges are held, and that deep massage in these zones will take away the negative charges—sort of deprogram the body."

"What kind of zones?"

"We got only to my face, but the scalp, for example, is concerned with worry." I look at her uneasily. "You see?"

"I don't see at all, but go on."

"Well, every part of the face is the psychic repository of emotion. The eyebrows hold anger, the forehead concern, the muscles around the eyes are prejudice, the nose external control, the part under the eyes shame, the lines on either side of the mouth disappointment, the ears the fear of not understanding, the chin inferiority . . ."

"Do you know what I think?"

"I think I'd rather tell you the rest," I say quickly. "When there's a trauma to any part of the body, the body doesn't like to remember it. The mind turns off and desensitizes that area. You feel it less, as if it were anesthetized. Once you begin to massage that area with *Chua-ka*, you have to put the same amount of energy into it as it lost. Do you understand?"

"No. It doesn't make any sense at all. Tell me about the massage."

"The goal of *Chua-ka*, as Bob explained it to me, is to be able to touch any bone in the body without pain."

"Any bone?"

"It's deep massage, on the borderline between pleasure and pain. It gives you a supple sort of strength."

"You're losing me again. How is it done?"

"With the fingertips and with small instruments made of bone or ivory or plastic. You see, the body accumulates karma."

"Karma?"

"That's everything that separates us from reality. This karma has a physiological manifestation in the body, little fatty globules that accumulate. Normally, they would be circulating energy." At her bewildered look, I hurry along, repeating Bob's involved pitch. "One of the effects of the massage is to break up these fatty globules."

"Why not?"

"I'll tell you what happened, straight. I went to Bob's apartment for the *Chua-ka*, and after this involved explanation, I stretched out on a pad on the floor and . . ."

"No table?" My wife interrupts.

I look pained. "Please. No table, no chairs, no bed, no desk—just pads and pillows all over the floor. He takes the lotus position behind me, puts a pillow on his lap, and I lie on my back with the pillow under my head. Then he plays a record on his stereo."

"Music too! What record?"

"A very monotonous sort of chant. The words 'I am consciousness' repeated again and again, ad infinitum—or ad a half hour. He called it a repetition. It was curious. Then he began to knead my face. He would find the insertion of each muscle and press in with a great deal of strength. It really was on that thin edge between pain and pleasure. He started with my jaw muscles, and then moved out to my ocular orbits, the muscles around my mouth, my forehead, my nose . . ."

"I can see what happened there. It's black and blue."

"A little too much pressure. Then my ears. I dozed off while he was doing my ears."

"How could you, if it hurt?"

"Well, it didn't hurt that much. But I'll tell you a curious thing. If you cut away all the nonsensical explanation of the method and just consider the deep massage of my facial muscles with his fingers and that ivory *ka*, his instrument, a funny thing happened. I experienced a strange, hypnotic high."

"Are you sure it wasn't the chanting?"

"That was part of it, but for about ten minutes before I fell asleep, I was really floating—the strangest, most pleasant sensation, and I think it was all a part of the rhythmic probing of my face."

"What was this high like?"

I frown a little and close my eyes, trying to remember. "I suddenly felt very euphoric, almost as if I were floating. I had my sense of time suspended. Later, Bob told me my face looked rhapsodic—as if I were off in another world. I had a subjective sensation of things stretched out indefinitely, the strangest feeling. Then I must have gone from that state to sleep. I slept for a minute or two and then came wide-awake."

"You called it strange. But was it good?"

"Yes, good enough so that I'd do it over again. That euphoric state lasted—even after I left the apartment. It was a raw, rainy day outside, but I hardly felt the weather, I had such a deep glow."

"Well, then, it must have been a success."

"Oh, yes, in terms of feeling good. I don't know about the karma and fat globules and the rest of the mystical rigmarole, but if the Genghis Khan story is true, I could see how a tired warrior could be recharged for battle."

"But he only did your face."

"For over an hour. The next session is another hour, and then he does the feet. Then there's a session for each side of the body. He likes to give you a session a week. I may go back for another one—as soon as I decide which part of my body needs it most."

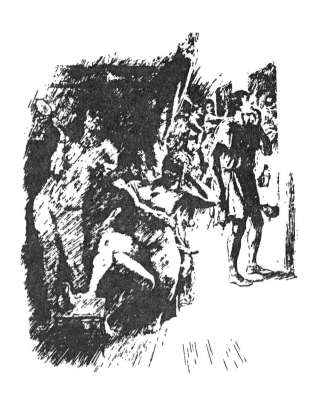

THE SWING
OF THINGS

Have you ever wondered what kind of people are "swingers"? I talked with three couples who challenged my preconceptions in a most pleasant way.

The evening starts like any other social get-together: three couples sitting around my living room with drinks, very ordinary-looking couples in their late twenties or early thirties. But there is a difference, and the difference makes me a shade uneasy. All of these couples belong to a national fraternity—they are swingers.

They have all agreed to an interview provided I use no names or identifying features—and indeed, looking at them, I realize how hard it would be to identify or characterize them.

They are all bland, ordinary, next-door-neighbor types, neither urban nor suburban in appearance, prototypes of the average American.

"One thing I want to ask you," I say. "Do you feel there's a difference between love and sex?"

There's a long pause while all of them smile, then one of the women says, "They really have nothing to do with each other, have they? I love my husband, and sex with him is wonderful, but I have sex with my friends, too, sometimes with men I've just met—and I don't love them. Oh, perhaps I love my friends, but in a different way, and there's no love at all with some of the men I have sex with."

Her husband nods. "You have to separate the physical from the emotional. You don't have to fall in love with a woman just because sex with her was great—not if you're all together."

"That's just it," another husband adds. "Being all together. We feel that we swingers are much more together, more complete than traditional married couples. Sure, we've got children, jobs—we're like anyone else—but swinging is a very special kind of thing with us. It opens us up."

"It's honest," his wife joins in. "It's not like—well, before I married, when I was still dating, everything was a charade. I had to play the part of the shy female. The guy was the aggressive male. Even in bed we kept the same roles. We played games."

"And now?"

She shrugs. "There's no longer any need to play games. I have so much choice. No one has to prove anything with us. If things don't work out with one partner, you try another—and both of you are relaxed. There's no sense of performance."

"This swinging," I ask. "Is it done at home—in parties? What about your children?"

"What about them?" another wife says with a little frown. "I make sure that mine have no part of the swinging scene. They're only seven and nine years old—too young to understand. When I give a swinging party, I pack them off to grandma. If I go to one, I have a baby-sitter in. But then, you wouldn't have kids in any adult get-together, would you?"

"Tell me a little about swinging," I ask. "When it comes right down to it, I don't really know what goes on at a swingers' get together. Is it wife swapping?"

One of the women shakes her head. "I hate that. It sounds as if we were—well, objects that husbands have the right to trade! You never hear about husband swapping."

One of the husbands says, "You know, swinging isn't just trading mates. If anything could describe it, it would be sexual freedom. We get together—say three, four, or five couples—and we feel free to have sex—or not to have it."

"What happens at a typical party?"

"No party's typical. They all vary," he answers slowly. "Like a party we went to last week. Most of the guests were married couples we knew; a few were strangers. The house was nicely decorated with soft lights. We sat around for a while. Then I saw a woman I liked, and I smiled at her. We talked for a while, and then I just took her hand and led her into the bedroom. We stripped and went to bed together."

"Just like that?"

"Of course. There was no need for hypocrisy. We both knew why we were there, and she was free to say no. She knew I wouldn't be offended."

I turn to his wife. "Were you upset?"

She laughs. "Why should I have been. I wandered into the bedroom and watched them for a while, and then someone came in behind me. He began to make love to me while we were watching, and then we both got undressed and joined them."

"It was a king-sized bed!" her husband laughs.

"And you weren't at all jealous, seeing your husband with another woman?"

Again she laughs. "Not a bit. I was pleased that he was finding pleasure with another woman, and, quite frankly, I was excited—so excited that I joined him with another man."

"A stranger?"

She shrugs. "What's the difference? I knew everybody at the party. I was willing to have sex with anyone there."

"In any arrangement?"

There's a moment's hesitation, and then she says, "If you mean with another woman, yes. I've done that and enjoyed it."

"And how would you feel about sex with another man?" I ask her husband.

He shakes his head with hesitation. "I'm not into that scene!"

"I've never run into two men making it," one of the other husbands says slowly. "Women, yes—but men—it's just not—well, not what swingers do."

The third husband says, "Two women making it turn me on. But two men don't turn a woman on."

Letting that go, I ask, "Isn't there a tremendous preoccupation with sex among swingers? From what many of you say I get the impression that your parties all revolve around sex."

He shakes his head. "Not true at all. Sure, our swinging parties revolve around sex, but we have plenty of other social get-togethers, and we have straight friends, nonswingers. For God's sake, you know, it's the nonswingers who have this preoccupation with sex. Single guys who don't swing are always tuned in to who they're gonna date and whether they'll score with her—it takes all their energy. We don't worry about that. We know we can have as much sex as we want, whether we're married or single."

"What you have to keep in mind," one of the women says, leaning forward, "is that swinging can make a woman appreciate herself. It can make her realize that she's still sexually desirable. If she's locked into sex only with her husband, how will she ever know when he gets tired of her? What choices does he have?"

"Yes," her husband adds. "And if he does get tired, there's variety at any swingers' party. Swinging avoids just that, getting satiated with one partner."

"You've always got the option of someone else," another husband puts in.

"And it's sex, not love, we're talking about," his wife adds. "You can love your husband and still be tired of sex with him alone."

"Aren't there problems inherent in the life-style of the swinger?" I ask after a moment's thought.

"Oh, sure," a wife says quickly. "We've run into the problem of disapproving neighbors. In fact, it once got so bad we had to move."

"And it wasn't that our parties were noisy," her husband adds. "It's just that our neighbors were very nosy and very puritanical."

"And your children? Do they know?"

There's a brief silence, then one of the women says, "My teen-age daughter has her suspicions, and I think, when she's old enough, she'll understand."

"I told my daughter. She's fifteen," one of the women says quietly.

"Did she understand?"

She shrugs. "I'm sure she did. She asked me so many questions about it, and finally her attitude was, 'If it's what you want to do and it doesn't hurt anyone—why not?' She pauses a moment. "But I think the biggest impression she got from our talk was, 'My mother was honest with me. She trusted me.' You know, that talk made us both very close."

"My children are too young," the third wife says. "We hide it from them, and that's right for us. I don't think I could ever tell them." She smiles at the others. "That takes a kind of bravery I just don't have."

"Someday you'll tell them," one of the husbands assures her. "And you'll find it isn't too bad." He frowns a bit. "You know, I've been thinking, all through this discussion, one of the positive things about swinging is the lack of emasculating women in the scene."

"What do you mean?"

"Well, in most sexual relationships you find that women resent the whole setup, and many of them react by trying to 'get' the man. That isn't true with swingers. Swinging women seem to wake up to their own sexuality, to enjoy sex more. It all becomes less threatening, more casual, not such a big deal. That's another point in answer to what you said before. Once we start swinging, sex stops dominating our lives."

"I'd think it would be just the opposite."

"Not at all. It's there, it's available, so why make a big fuss about it? Once we relax about the whole sexual scene, once we can dispel our hang-ups about it, we can get onto the other important aspects of life."

"Like a good cup of coffee," another husband says with a grin. "Did you offer us some? I could really use it."

We all laugh as I turn off my tape recorder.

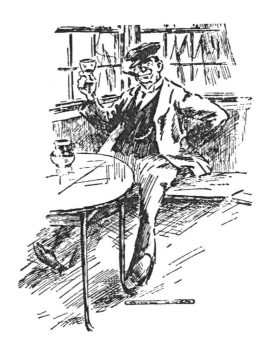

I WAS A JUNK-FOOD JUNKIE

Has the junk-food urge ruined every diet you've tried? You can kick the habit. All it takes is some basic changes in where and how you eat.

"OhmiGawd!" Burt cries out in anguish as he pulls over to the right-hand lane. "Stop me before it's too late!"

"What's wrong?" I ask, alarmed. I've been dozing lightly while Burt drove, and now I'm suddenly awake, my heart racing, my body braced against the expected shock of an accident. "Are we all right?"

The road is clear, but Burt's teeth are clenched, his brow creased. "It's coming up and I can't resist!"

"What the hell are you talking about? Is anything wrong with the car? What is it, a flat?"

He's slowed down considerably, and he gestures ahead at the elaborate logo of a nationally famous hamburger joint looming above the highway. "It's my nemesis. You didn't know when we started this trip—I didn't have the courage to tell you—but I'm a junk-food junkie."

"A what?" It's some kind of a gag, I realize, and I settle back in my seat, my pulse still racing. "I could gladly break your head in four pieces," I say grimly. "I'm too old for this nonsense!"

"Nonsense, he calls it!" Burt turns innocent twenty-two-year-old eyes on me. "It's a matter of life and breadth. I'm overweight, too fat for the tennis court. I'm beginning to move like Frankenstein's monster, and you tell me it's nonsense!"

He pulls into the hamburger joint's parking lot and he turns toward me, his face stricken. "I'm very serious. I've put on so much weight in the last year, since college and this new job, that it's like a disease."

"You mean gaining weight?"

"How I gain it. I'm very troubled. I'm really a junk-food junkie. It started in college, and now I can't resist it. I fill up on junk food constantly. French fries kill me, and I'm mad for potato chips. Soft drinks, candy bars—and cookies! Wow! I can kill a box of Oreos in no time flat. I go on jelly-bean busts—I freak out on them. I've been known to buy two or three pounds, go to a movie theater, and eat them one by one in the dark. Three pounds will see me through a full-length feature—if I nurse them a bit."

"You don't feel sick afterward?"

"I think—I'm not sure, but I think that I get something like sugar poisoning."

"Hyperglycemia?"

"That sounds pretty bad. My heart races, and I feel sick and dizzy. I almost pass out."

"Then why do it?"

Burt throws up his arms. "Why do it? Ask a junkie why take heroin when he knows it destroys him. I'm hooked on junk foods. Crackerjacks! I have a closet full. When my mother comes to see my apartment, I have to hide them in all the spots I think she won't check—and for a mother, that's not many. In my typewriter case, under the dirty clothes in the hamper, in plastic bags in the toilet box . . ."

"You're putting me on!"

We get out of the car and Burt shakes his head. "Just a little. It's a terrible thing, though. I just *must* lose weight before the summer. I'm ashamed to be seen on the beach looking like this, but what can I do? I can't resist junk food, and these places are all along the road—or maybe I'm just out on the road more often."

As we sit down and Burt looks at the menu glumly, I tell him, "This kind of eating place can be a catastrophe, you know that?"

"How well I know it! Look at this menu. A three-decker hamburger. I'd give my eyetooth for that."

"It has to be at least 600 calories."

He shakes his head somberly. "And a chocolate shake? Is that too bad?"

"I'd say over 300 calories."

"What about a small order of french fries? A small one?"

"Would you believe 250 calories? If they're not greasy."

"I like them greasy. And that hot apple pie? It looks good enough to eat!"

"It is, but without that little wedge of cheese it's easily 450 calories. Burt! That's more than 1,500 calories for lunch alone. No wonder you're getting fatter every time I see you."

With a touch of despair, he says, "I tell you what. You order for me. You'll see. There's no way out."

"You can't cook your own food?"

"I'm on the road too much. Seriously now, I could manage to control my junkie tastes at home, get rid of all the Crackerjacks and candy bars, but what good would that do? You know I have to travel on the job. I'm always on the move, driving my own car or a rented one. I eat all my meals out, so what can I do?"

"First off—resist these fast-food traps."

"Should we walk out now?" He looks woebegone and I laugh.

"No. Let's see if you can order sensibly, even here. Let's cut out the hamburger bun. All it docs is add calories. Without the bun, or the double decker, a quarter pound of hamburger, if it's lean, should be a shade over 300 calories. That's not bad because a lot of it is protein. If you want to fancy it up, order it with cheese. That'll make it 400, and a few more for catsup and pickles—maybe 450 altogether."

"And french fries?" he says wistfully.

"If you're hooked, order a small portion, but—you get to eat only half. Throw the rest away before you start. You can get away with 110 calories."

"So we're up to, let's see, 560?" he asks hopefully.

"That's right. No milkshake."

"What? Not even half?"

"Junk food! You go cold turkey. Diet soda—and no pie. You see those apples on the counter? Ask for one."

"They're probably only for decoration."

"You have to face reality," I tell him firmly. "From now on, dessert is an apple or an orange or maybe a pear. If you can't buy it, then carry a bag with you in the car when you travel and have your dessert when you leave the restaurant."

The waitress comes and we order, Burt asking for a plain hamburger without the bun. "I can't do that," the waitress tells him. "You gotta take it the way it comes."

"Throw the bun away," I tell him as his face lights up. He sighs and agrees, and when his order comes, he discards the bun and half the french fries.

"You think this will take off weight?"

"Well, look at the calories. With the apple we'll snitch from the display, it's still less than 700 calories, less than half of what you would have had. Even if you don't lose weight, you won't gain as much as you did."

Burt eats thoughtfully, and when we leave the hamburger
joint to finish our ride, he's very quiet. "I want to thank you,"
he says thoughtfully when we say good-bye that afternoon.
"You've started me thinking."

I don't realize how serious Burt is until I meet him two
months later at a friend's house. To my amazement, he's lost
almost all the extra poundage he had put on with his new job.
"You look great," I tell him.

"I *am* great," he grins. "I've licked the junk food habit
single-handed—well, maybe not single-handed. You gave me a
boost, but you know, I learned something that day."

"What?"

"I learned that you can arrange your life the way you want
it, no matter what the circumstances."

"That's pretty heavy stuff."

"No, listen. I still have the same job. I travel as much as
ever, and I eat out constantly—but I've learned the rules."

"Which are?"

"Well, for one thing, I plan ahead. I know exactly what I'm
going to eat when I hit a restaurant. I don't look at the menu. I
ask, 'Have you a nice piece of broiled fish, or lean meat or
chicken. Give me a green vegetable and a salad. Oil and
vinegar, and I'll put it on myself.' Then I say, 'Bring me a glass
of tomato juice right away,' or I ask for a half grapefruit or a
cup of tea or coffee if it's cold out."

"What does that do?"

"It keeps me from devouring the bread—you know those
baskets of rolls or fresh bread they put out?"

"Not at hamburger joints."

"I don't eat there anymore. Only good restaurants. And I
take your advice and carry a bag of apples in the car. I have
one before dinner, a half hour or so before. That takes the
edge off my appetite."

"Anything else?"

He shrugs. "Common sense. I eat slowly, very slowly. I've
given up desserts except for melons and fruits cups. In short—
I'm no longer a junk-food junkie. I can drive past the golden

arches, the Colonel's bucket, the hamburger heavens, and all the others. I think I'm growing up."

"I shouldn't be surprised," I tell him, and I pat his stomach. "At least you're not growing out!"

> *Staying out of the hamburger joints will help, but not if you go next door to a quality restaurant and gorge yourself. Follow Burt's example and be careful about what you eat even after you've kicked the junk-food habit.*

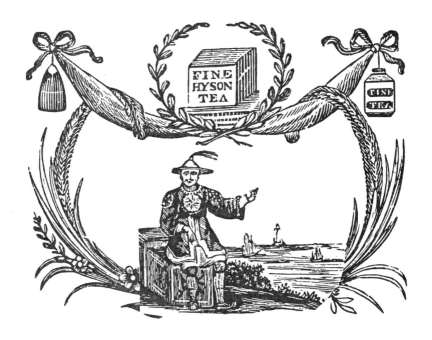

A CEREMONIAL
DELIGHT

When everything begins to seem ordinary and drab and uninteresting, maybe the problem is that your senses have become dulled. Here's a sensible way to bring your senses back to life.

I have met my friends, Martin, Beverly, and Okakura for tea at a downtown hotel. It's a winter afternoon, and we come from the cold, cheerless gray of the outside to the warm yellow lights of the hotel. Tea is served in a part of the lobby screened off from the rest by tall palms in pots and graceful hanging ferns. The table linen is white, the silver ornate, and the teacups surprisingly fragile for a hotel. A slender silver vase holds a full-blown chrysanthemum.

"Tea! I love it," Beverly says with a little sigh of content. "It's so civilized."

Okakura sips his tea and smiles. "A good drink. It hasn't the arrogance of wine, the self-consciousness of coffee, nor the simpering innocence of cocoa."

"What a wonderful description!" Martin says. "Yours?"

Reluctantly, Okakura says, "No. A namesake of mine who wrote a book on the tea ceremony used it first. That was back at the turn of the century. They looked at things differently then."

"Just what is the tea ceremony?" Beverly asks. "I've heard so much about it. Does it really raise your consciousness?"

Okakura is silent for a moment, smiling. Then he sighs. "How can I give you a quick history of tea? It is so much a part of my Japanese culture—and Chinese culture, too. You know, it used to be called 'tow.' Then, in the fourth or fifth century, the modern Chinese ideograph—which we Japanese use, too—was created, and it was called 'cha.' In modern times it's been compressed into 'tay' and 'tee' and here and now to 'tea.' "

"What's the right way to make it?" Beverly asks.

Okakura shrugs. "There is no right way. They used to steam the leaves, crush them in a mortar, and make them into a cake. That was many centuries ago. To brew it, they'd boil the cake with rice, orange peel, ginger—even onions!" He puts up his hand when we laugh. "No, it's true. And they still make it that way in parts of Tibet and Mongolia."

Martin grimaces. "It sounds wild, and it must taste awful."

"Well, the Russians still add lemon to tea, and that custom has taken hold here. We Japanese think that's pretty awful. The English, who took to tea like ducks to water, add milk to theirs, and I think they're both barbarous practices. You know, the early method of brewing tea changed in the Tang dynasty. Then they powdered the leaves and added hot water and whipped it to a froth with bamboo whisks. The Ming dynasty brought about our modern method of tea making, steeping the leaves in hot water. But modern China has let the mystique about tea disappear, and Japan has taken it up."

He shakes his head thoughtfully. "With us, tea drinking

became a religion of the art of life, a way to worship purity and refinement, an improvised drama."

We are all quiet for a few moments, then Martin says, "But tell us more about the tea ceremony."

"Basically," Okakura says thoughtfully, "it's a development of the Zen ritual. Zen, you know, is the successor of Taoism."

We nod, though none of us knew it till then.

"Taoism, of course," Okakura continues, "contributed most to aesthetics. Zen emphasizes the teachings of Taoism. It holds that the ultimate in self-realization can be obtained from meditation." He frowns a bit. "Let me put it this way. Zen aims at direct communion with the inner nature of things. It regards the outer forms as blocks to the perception of truths."

"But as far as tea is concerned . . ." Beverly prompts.

"Well, I just wanted to give you an impression of Zen thinking. Now, for the drinking of tea. The first necessity is the proper surrounding. In Japan we build special tea rooms— or we used to when life was slower and more elegant. The rooms weren't lavish. Indeed, they are intended to give an impression of refined poverty. The room should be simple and pure, like a Zen monastery. The orthodox tea room is about ten feet square, and it's built out in the garden. The path to the room is extremely important. It should give an impression of serenity and purity. You know, the door to an orthodox tea room is only three feet high so that you must bend low to enter. That teaches humility."

Beverly looks around at the soft lights of the hotel. "And this as a substitute . . ."

Okakura sighs. "Space is nonexistent to the truly enlightened. This is an admirable substitute, but usually the tea room is very empty. A flower arrangement, one priceless vase—enough! And there is the kettle, and the teapot, the pitcher, the cups. All should be different.

"We come into the tea room and first we appreciate the art, the flowers, the vase, the teacups—the one exquisite object of art in the teahouse." He lifts a hotel teacup and touches it with his fingers. "It may be the teacup itself, so fragile it seems made of foam, so delicately glazed and colored, or the beautiful object may be a flower arrangement, or even one blossom in a perfect setting."

"But the ceremony?" Martin asks impatiently.

"Oh?" Okakura says in some surprise. "But I have been giving you the ceremony all along. There is left only the pouring and the sipping of the tea, but all the rest, the serenity of mind, the quality of conversation, the principles of Zen, the appreciation of the room, the art—this is all part of the tea ceremony."

"And what does it do?"

"Do? It is not a ceremony that *does* something. It is a way of opening the mind, embracing the inner sight, a way of educating the senses." Okakura pours another cup of tea from the pot and he shudders as he reaches inside and removes three teabags. "There is tea and there is tea—but even so." He lifts his cup and savors the aroma, then sips the tea slowly.

"You must understand that everything about the tea ceremony is designed to open your eyes to beauty, to cleanse your senses. That is the Zen of it." He looks around the hotel lobby. "Now even here there is beauty in the soft lights, the polished brass, the linen and silver, in the lovely dresses of the ladies, in the occasional elegant turn of the nape of someone's neck, a beauty you can understand and appreciate as you drink your tea. Even the flowers." He touches the chrysanthemum in the vase. "Its shape is exquisite, a joy to the eye."

I sip at my cup and nod. "I think I understand. It's a ceremony to open our eyes, to see just a bit differently, even if what we see is ordinary."

"Exactly. There is beauty all around us, always. We must be trained to observe it."

Beverly raises her cup, "I'll drink to that!" And we all do, very solemnly.

> *Supermarket tea is adequate—if you can't find anything else. But it's well worth your while to buy your tea from a Chinese or Japanese specialty food store. Experiment a little. You may be surprised at some of the exotic flavors you'll find.*

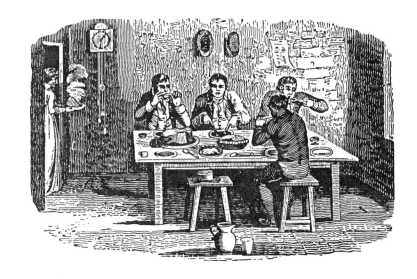

WHY WE WANT
TO EAT—AND ONE
POSSIBLE SOLUTION

Your "hunger mechanism" is what makes you want to eat. Some medical researchers I know have some fascinating ideas about ways to turn off that "mechanism."

"Why do I get hungry?" I asked David.

"That's an intriguing question," he said with a smile. "How am I to answer it?"

David, an intern in a large New York hospital, had brought his friend Anita to meet Sally, a research student visiting us from Cambridge. Stubbing out her cigarette, Anita said, "It's like you men to ask and answer those silly questions. You get hungry because you haven't eaten."

"Ah, but that's the point," I said quickly. "I can sometimes go for most of the day without eating and still not feel hungry. Then something will trigger my appetite, and all at once I'm ravenous—or I can finish a meal and an hour later feel hungry again."

In her delightful English accent, Sally said, "Perhaps your mouth was the culprit."

David looked at her sharply. "But isn't it the hypothalamus that controls appetite? We've been taught that when different parts of the hypothalamus are destroyed, there are profound effects on eating habits."

"What effects?" Anita asked.

"Well—paradoxical effects, in a way, yet logical ones. I remember reading about experiments with rats. Destroying one part turned the rat into a compulsive eater. Destroying another part made him refuse to eat—in fact, he starved to death!"

Anita shivered. "What a gruesome thing! Could that be why some of us are fat and some are thin? I mean, could we have damaged our hypothalamuses—or is it hypothalami?"

"I don't agree with you, David," Sally said with a little frown. "Dr. Zeigler, who worked with birds at Cambridge, found that when you damaged the brain, a good distance from the hypothalamus, the birds still stopped eating."

But they were birds," David smiled. "We may be bird-brained, but we're human."

Sally shook her head. "Let me tell you the whole story. Dr. Zeigler spoke about his work to an anatomist at the Massachusetts Institute of Technology. This man told him that the part of the brain damaged in his birds received information from the same nerve network that brought touch, temperature, and pain from the mouth to the brain. Do you get the point?"

I said, "Do you mean that the part of the brain that tells us we're hungry also tells us about touch, temperature, and pain?"

"Yes, and it's not the hypothalamus."

"That's fascinating," David said. "Was there more to his work?"

"Well, yes. He went on to work with a neurophysiologist and study individual cells in that same nerve complex. They found that the cells responded to stimulation of different parts of the head and also to the opening and closing of the mouth."

"But what does it all mean?" Anita asked.

"Several things. Birds who suffer a lot of damage to that nerve complex stop eating for months."

"How do they live?"

"They fed them by tubes. Birds with less damage stopped eating for days, but even a lot of damage to the hypothalamus alone didn't affect eating. Only damage to that nerve complex made them starve."

"What was the complex called?" I asked.

"The trigeminal pathway. Those bird experts—I think they used pigeons—convinced Dr. Zeigler that damage to the trigeminal system got rid of hunger by getting rid of all oral stimulation."

"I have a very far-out idea," Anita said, her eyes wide. "If a drug could depress the trigeminal system, wouldn't it cause us to lose our appetites, to stop eating and take off weight?"

"My God," I said, impressed, "the drug companies would go mad over something like that. You could write your own ticket."

"But go ahead, Sally," David urged. "I'm fascinated by this work with birds. There's only one thing—could the researchers have damaged another part of the birds' brains when they were fooling around with the trigeminal system?"

"Well, that did occur to Dr. Zeigler. He cut the trigeminal nerve after it left the brain. That eliminated all feelings of touch and temperature—and the birds stopped eating. That seemed to prove that you need oral sensation to keep eating—at least in pigeons."

"But still, other animal work shows that destruction of the hypothalamus also causes loss of appetite," David said slowly.

"But that's just the point," Sally told him earnestly. "In most lab animals you can't destroy the hypothalamus without destroying the trigeminal nerve as well. Dr. Zeigler worked with rats after the birds and got the same results. Destroy the trigeminal nerve and you destroy the appetite."

"Are you saying the brain doesn't influence hunger?" David asked.

"Oh, no, only that the hypothalamus isn't the most important hunger-maker. We must think in terms of brain circuits instead of brain centers. The messages the body gets from inside, from the sugar or minerals in your blood, are important, but so are the outside messages."

"What are they?" Anita asked.

Sally spread her hands. "Chewing, swallowing, sucking—all of those arouse our appetite."

"Next to vision, touch is our most important sense," David said thoughtfully.

"Yes, and you know that the trigeminal system controls oral touch. The feel of Jell-O or ice cream or chocolate pudding has an effect on our eating habits."

"We sure are oral beings," Anita agreed. "Look how much nail biting, kissing, and chewing gum we all do."

"We start by sucking our thumb," David nodded.

"Now, it's possible, and this is the kicker," Sally said, sitting back with a smile, "that fat people need more oral stimulation, or they're more sensitive to it. They may eat normal meals, but they gain weight because they keep nibbling all day."

"Then what's the answer?" Anita asked. "The drug I thought of?"

"The answer should be simple. Find a sensual food with no food value, something a person can nibble all the time."

"Celery!" Anita clapped her hands with delight. "I love the crisp crunch of it, and it has almost no calories. How about a celery-nibbling diet?"

"Not bad," I said, "but my sensual kick in foods is smoother. Puddings or Jell-O or gumdrops."

"Then for you," Anita said, "it's gumdrops made of gelatin and artificial sweetener and food color to stimulate your eyes."

"I'd like that!" I agreed.

"For me," Sally laughed, "it's ice cream, but I'd substitute apple slush."

"What's that?"

"My father used to make it for me when I was a teen-ager. You cut up an apple and put orange juice and skim milk with it in a blender then add small ice cubes till it's mush. The calories are low, and the bulk is tremendous—and it tickles the palate."

"I'll take herb tea," Anita decided. "I could sip it all day, and it would satisfy my craving for oral stimulation."

"What I like," David nodded, "is fresh caviar. I could diet happily if I were as rich as an oil sheik and could nibble it all day and pop those fish eggs with my teeth. Wow!"

"No good," I told him regretfully. "It's about 90 calories an ounce."

He sighed. "Everything good is fattening or expensive, and caviar, naturally, is both. Well, that's the way the nibble goes."

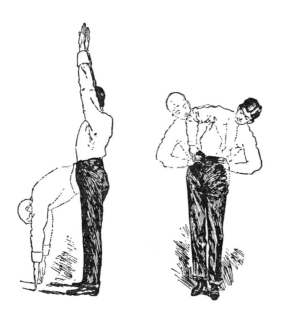

STANDING UP
TO THE PRESSURES
OF LIFE

This exercise plan hardly seems like exercise at all—until you find out how much good it does.

"Did you ever hear of the Comstock Laws?"

I look at Bill curiously and nod. "Sort of blue laws, weren't they? Something around the turn of the century?"

"Terribly puritanical. If a publisher printed a book with the picture of an unclothed body, he risked a year in jail and a thousand-dollar fine—and a thousand dollars was quite a lot in those days."

I say, "That's pretty sad, but they've been repealed for almost fifty years, haven't they? What have they got to do with us?"

"Well, the point is, if they hadn't been in existence, Dr. Mensendieck would have introduced her method of exercise into the United States in 1905 instead of having to take it to the Nordic countries, and we might all know about the method and use it, instead of it being such a mystery."

"To tell the truth, Bill, it's still a mystery to me. What the hell is this—Mensodict system?"

"Mensendieck," he corrects me. "It's a system of exercise that concentrates on correct and graceful body movements."

"What did it have to do with the Comstock laws?"

"Well, it couldn't be properly explained without nude pictures, and that was it. It's a shame because the method can not only bring a better function to the body, but it can also relieve pain."

"But how?"

"Well, you know, things like flat feet, bowed legs, sway back, potbelly, and even the dowager's hump that some women get after menopause aren't natural to the body. They develop from misuse. Bess Mensendieck showed how to use the body properly and avoid things like that. The primary part of her method is posture. She was a sculptor originally and then she became a physician. She stressed the fact that we all need to maintain proper posture during our everyday activities. That's the heart of her method."

"Is she dead now?"

"She died in her late nineties, hale and hearty!"

"Now you interest me. Tell me about her method."

"What can I tell you in the time we have?" Bill spreads his hands, then shrugs. "I'll try. Take the simple fact of standing. You should never toe out. Stand with your feet parallel. Turn in your buttocks and contract your abdominal muscles upward, then let your knee joints bend slightly. There! How does that feel?"

"A bit awkward."

"Now draw your shoulders back and down using the muscles in the middle of your back. Pull your neck up and rest your head on the top of your spine. Your elbows should be straight and the palms of your hands facing back. How's that?"

"Well—a bit strange. I'm not used to this posture. It pulls a lot of muscles into different shapes."

"You keep working at that posture and you'll feel better, much better. That's the basic stance of Mensendieck. Now, when you're walking, you keep that alignment. By pushing in your buttocks when you're keeping your body tall, you push your weight forward, and walking becomes easier."

I try walking that way for a while and agree that it's different. "But I'm not sure it's better."

"Because your back is twisted into its old alignment. Feeling better will come after a while. The next Mensendieck exercise is breathing. You breathe in through your nose and out through your mouth. When you inhale, try to use the muscles that expand the middle part of your lungs backward and sideways. When you exhale, let your lower ribs sag."

I practice Bill's method for a while, but I find that I'm growing light-headed. "Hyperventilation." Bill nods. "You're taking in more air than you're used to. You have to watch that. Now let me give you a few ways to do ordinary things in the Mensendieck method, like bending down to pick something up."

"Oh, I know about that," I tell him. "I bend my knees when I do it."

"No, this is when you have to reach forward and down. The trick is to limit the bending to the lower part of your body. That stretches the lower muscles. You tighten your abdominal muscles and bend only the five lumbar vertebrae."

I try it, shaking my head. "Now, that's going to take a lot of practice!"

"Well, sure. Who said it wouldn't? Now you spoke of stooping by bending your knees. When you do that, you have to tighten the muscles around your pelvis. Pull your abdomen up and your buttocks together and down, and while you're doing that, bend your knees straight forward, as deeply as possible. You see, instead of letting your weight bend you, you make your muscles bend your body."

"I think I've got it," I say as I lower and raise my body, "But it's difficult."

"All of the Mensendieck method is. Even sitting down and

getting up is difficult—at first. You use your buttock muscles to sit and stand. You stabilize your pelvis by tensing all the muscles around it; then you bend your knees and your lower vertebrae. When you touch the chair seat, you straighten your back and release your buttock muscles."

"I can see that you're concentrating on using the muscles to support the body."

"Exactly! You do it even when you're sitting. You should be erect, using your muscles to support you instead of relying completely on the chair and table. And it carries over to all aspects of moving. Look. To pick something up, I bend my knees and my lumbar vertebrae, then lift myself up with my buttock muscles. I'm really using my back."

I try to see the distinction as I pick something up the old way and the new Mensendieck way. Mostly I feel that the difference is postural, but Bill assures me it's also muscular. To lift a weight, he tightens his pelvic muscles, exhaling, and contracts his abdominal muscles, then lifts. "You see," he explains, "this allows the center of your body—the real source of body power—to do the lifting, when you do anything—say go up and down stairs—keep erect. Climb on your forward leg and let it lift you. Go down stairs by doing a knee bend with your back leg. Let it lower you."

To kneel, Bill explains, you still use your buttocks, lifting your trunk forward and up while a knee bend lowers your back knee to the floor, then follow it with the other knee. "And always," he emphasizes, "walk with your body weight ahead of your parallel feet. Keep your pelvic muscles tense, and you'll feel as if your abdomen and buttocks are doing the work instead of your legs."

Watching him, I'm impressed with a certain grace and dignity about his posture. I've seen a few of the old Hollywood stars move like that, an erect, confident movement. I try to imitate it, following Bill's directions, but it becomes too much of a strain for me and I lapse back into my old, comfortable stance.

"You have to work at it," Bill assures me. "There are plenty of books about the Mensendieck method, and you ought to get one and practice the exercises. You'll see a remarkable change in your posture."

The thought of a regular routine of exercises is dismal, but Bill reassures me. "Once you get into the swing of it, it's all cake, and it's not only posture correction that's so great about it, it can be used in training for childbirth and reconditioning your body after an accident. It's terrific for actors and dancers, and you know—it's not strenuous. Cardiac and orthopedic patients can do the exercises. It's just—" He bites his lip and frowns. "Well, a reconditioning of your body."

I like that, I tell Bill. "Let me practice what you've shown me, and if it works out, I'll look up the exercises. I leave him and I walk away erect, trying to keep my feet parallel, my buttocks tense and my head up. It's not quite as hard as I thought, and I decide my first stop on the way home is the public library to look up a few books by Dr. Elizabeth Mensendieck.

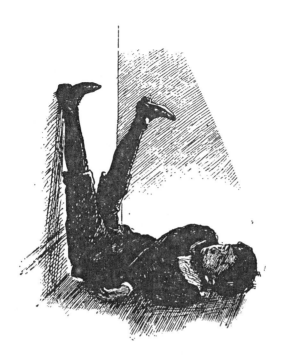

EXERCISE
YOUR BODY
AND MIND

Here's an exercise program that can help you feel good mentally as it builds up your body.

Robin and Moira, pretty, vivacious and still in their twenties are visiting us from the West Coast, and both are delighted and disappointed with New York City. "There's so much to do," Robin tells me, "but you New Yorkers forget the inner life."

"If it weren't for psychocalisthenics," Moira adds, "I don't think we could survive here for a whole week."

That fascinates me. "What are psychocalisthenics?"

"They're a series of exercises that you do in sequence, and they work out every part of your body."

"But any good set of exercises does that," I protest.

"Well, psychocalisthenics is more than just a set of exercises," Robin puts in. "There are breathing exercises that go with each body exercise, and together they create a state of well-being that's mental as well as physical."

"Let me show you," Moira says, lying down on the floor on her back. She lifts her feet and buttocks, slips her hands onto the small of her back, and suddenly she's standing on her head. She sways for a breathless moment, then steadies herself.

"We start with the headstand." Robin explains.

I watch Moira's face become a pleasant pink. "In the morning?"

"Right after we get up—after our meditation, of course."

Moira slips down on her back and then jumps to her feet. "Between each exercise, we breathe deeply." Suiting her actions to her words, she says, "I clasp my hands in front of me and raise them over my head as I inhale. I hold that breath to the count of three, then exhale as I lower my arms."

"Breathing opens you up," Robin nods. "It helps your circulation and calms you down."

"The point is," Moira adds, "as you exercise, you concentrate on that part of the body that you're moving. It's like meditation. You put your consciousness into that part of your body." She repeats the breathing exercise, her eyes closed. Then she opens them and smiles. "Now, while I did that, I concentrated on the cool air coming into my body, going down to my lungs and into my blood—then through my whole body." She spreads her hands benignly.

"In other words," Robin says, "you go along with whatever is happening in your body and in essence separate your mind from your body—the same as you do in transcendental meditation. Look, here's another exercise." She bends forward and puts her hands on the floor, her head down, then moves her feet forward till her body forms a pyramid. "Now I concentrate on the center of my body, about four fingers below my belly button. Then I straighten up slowly and finish with a breathing exercise."

"Here's another." Moira puts her feet about ten inches apart. "It's called 'Picking Grapes.' When you do it, honestly you can feel a surge of energy through your whole body." She bends her knees slightly, exhaling as she bends from the shoulders. Then she swings her arms up and reaches above her with each hand. "You exhale to the count of three, then breathe in again as you reach up."

"Here is another!" Robin reaches above her head, standing on her toes, then bends her back to one side, straightens up and then bends to the other, then she pulls her arms down and crouches. "It's called 'The Dancer.' You do it five times, exhaling on the crouch."

"We do most of the exercises five times," Moira adds. "You see, it's not to strengthen us or to limber us up—just to clean out our heads." The two of them, side by side, bend forward to touch the floor, then straighten, arms over heads, and arch their backs. "Inhale as you bend, exhale as you rise."

"Then there's 'The Ax.'" They bend at the hip, then lift their clasped hands to one side like a woodchopper and swing forward in a down stroke. "Exhale as you go down, inhale as you go up."

"Inhale through the nose and exhale through the mouth—always," Robin says as she straightens up from the Ax. "Every exercise has a name."

They demonstrate in a unison that puts me in mind of a Russian gymnast: the Shoulder Roll, with hands clasped behind their heads; the Crouch, bending at the knees with hands touching the ground; the Metronome, in which they extend their arms and swing from side to side; The Eggbeater, with hands twisting at the wrists; the Windmill (very good for the circulation—you can feel your fingers tingling!), with arms swinging around like the blades of a windmill; the Scythe, swinging locked hands from side to side; Head Rolls, which start by drooping the chin and rolling first clockwise, then counterclockwise; and the Camel, head backward, then forward—all with the inhale-exhale accompaniment.

There seems no end to the names and varieties of exercise, and I begin to feel exhausted watching them. They go into the

Shoulder Stand, lying on their backs and lifting their feet behind their heads; the Bow, on their buttocks with both arms reaching to touch their toes, legs and backs at an angle from the floor, their arms the bowstring. In the Scissors, they get into the bicycling position, but instead of peddling, scissor their feet. Then they ease up to the Cobra, on their stomachs as they lift their heads and chests.

They finish with Salute to the Sun, with their hands on their shoulders. They crouch, then touch fingers to the floor then rise, arms at their side, head lifted and chin pointed ahead, the whole done with an easy grace.

"And you tell me this isn't working out!"

Robin flings herself down on the floor and laughs while Moira, more serious, says, "The really important thing is to meditate as you do it. Then you can feel that surge of energy go through you."

"But how can you meditate when the exercises are so complex?"

"Well, that's just it. You take a series of these calisthenics, oh any sequence, and rehearse them to the point where they're automatic, then you run through them while you allow your mind to drift. That relaxes your mind while the exercise is relaxing your body."

"And it doesn't tire you?"

"Oh, no. It gives me this incredible energy and I'm ready for the day. You see, you pull in a lot of oxygen by breathing so deeply and that stimulates your brain."

"There's another thing," Robin says, sitting up abruptly. "This puts you in touch with your body. You feel every muscle, and that increased awareness makes your body come alive and you become a part of the world around you. You have a better relationship with other people."

"And you do this every morning?"

"Well ..." Robin laughs. "We should, but somehow it's hard. You know, it won't reshape your body but it sure as hell reshapes your mind."

"For me," Moira says thoughtfully, "I find that it alters my state of consciousness. Maybe it's the extra oxygen, but whatever—I feel that I'm on a different level, twice as alive. That's really it, that extra shot of life!"

This system illustrates an important lesson about any exercise plan: it should feel good. All worthwhile exercise programs will help you feel better in the long run, but if yours can give you a sense of well-being now—today—that's even better: your exercising will enrich your life as it builds up your body. And if you enjoy your exercise program, you will be more likely to stick with it long enough to make it work.

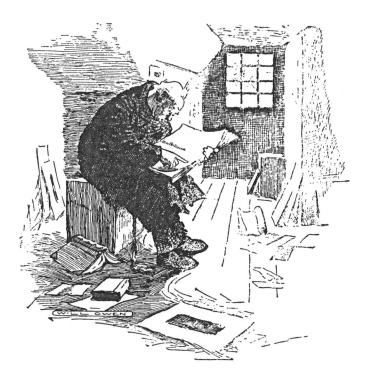

ADDING UP TO A LOSS

If you're good with details and want to go on a diet, I couldn't suggest a better one than the technique a friend of mine tried. This man's system has some good ideas for anyone who wants to lose weight.

"I have taken up 'The Bookkeeper's Diet,'" Ted declared.

I looked at him speculatively. "Evidently you've been balancing your books." When I last saw Ted, he topped the scales at an even 300 pounds. Now he was well below 250. This wasn't quite as bad as it sounds because Ted is 6'5", and he has a heavy frame. His normal weight is over 200. At 300 he was heavy, but he never seemed obese. He carried his fat with flair.

"But I felt it," he confessed to me as we sat over a cup of coffee at a roadside diner. "It began to be an effort just to get around, and in my racket I have to get around a lot."

Ted was a salesman for a data-processing company, and he was always on the road, touching home base only three or four times a week. "It played hell with my marriage—all this traveling," he told me, frowning down at his cup. "I guess that was the real reason Madge and I split up. She couldn't take an absentee husband. After the divorce, it got worse. I guess I just ate to comfort myself."

Grinning wryly, he adds. "That was when I discovered halvah and freaked out."

"Halvah?"

"Yeah. You know that Turkish candy made of sugar and egg white and sesame seeds and calories. You can get it in candy stores, packaged or sometimes covered with chocolate, but the real stuff comes in big tubs and only certain stores—usually in big cities—carry it. I'd hit a city when I was on the road and I'd search out the local halvah center before I even checked into my hotel. I'd buy a pound—a whole pound, for chrissakes—and I'd stretch out in bed, turn on the TV, and eat up a storm. I gained 75 pounds in six months of halvah orgies!"

Shaking my head in disbelief, I said, "Just on halvah?"

"Oh, that was my basic staple. I ate other things, believe me. I was on an expense account, and I'd have breakfast with eggs and bacon and hot cereal, and drinks with my dinner, wine, dessert, brandy—the whole *schtick*. I just jammed it all in. You know, it was like there was some terrible, empty void in me, and I had to fill it up." He signaled the waitress. "Can you toast me one of those corn muffins?"

For a minute he was quiet, watching the waitress. Then he said, "Now I think it was missing Madge. That was the emptiness in my life, and I tried to fill it with food."

"That sounds sort of simple."

"Simple or not, it was so. Oh, I'm an eater. I've always been. Some people run to fat, but I gallop. Still, I've always been able to keep it under control. With Madge gone, I just lost control."

"What did you mean by taking up 'The bookkeeper's diet'?"

"That's what I call it. I picked up the idea at the University of Pennsylvania when I was trying to sell a computer setup to their medical department. Some doctor there—I don't remember his name—had a long talk with me and told me about the weight clinic they run and how they help people like me. The big thing about it all, I gathered from what he said, was the record keeping."

"How did that work?"

"Well, I carried a little book around with me—a small ledger—and I treated it just like a bookkeeping problem. On the debit side I put down everything I ate every day—and I listed the calories. The doc gave me a list of calorie counts in every food, and I stapled it into the front of my ledger.

"I kept some set of books, let me tell you. I entered the time I ate, the place, who I was with, and what I had been doing. I'd go into detail, like when I lost a big sale to IBM out on the Coast and I promptly bought a half gallon of butter pecan ice cream and ate it all in my hotel room.

"I told myself I had to finish it to keep it from melting because I had no freezer. But in my bookkeeping I was honest. I put in a footnote that said, 'Who stood behind you with a gun and kept you from buying a pint, or even a quart?'

"The whole point of the notation was to let me know, not only how much I was eating and how fattening it all was—ice cream, halvah, cookies, candy bars, rich sauces, desserts and wines—but also why I ate."

"Not because you were hungry?"

"Sure, because I was hungry, but what caused that hunger? My body didn't need all that food. All it was doing was storing up fat, and what did I need it all for? I wasn't going into hibernation. Look, losing Madge was one thing, losing a sale, missing a plane, getting to a hotel and finding my room wasn't ready, or they had overbooked and I was without a place to stay—all the petty frustrations, and the big ones, aroused one reaction. Eat! Fill my face!

"I never realized how obvious the pattern was until I saw it all there in black and white, in debits and credits."

"What were the credits?"

"How I expended the calories. You know, for each pound I weigh, a guy like me, one who runs around the way I do, needs about 14 calories a day. So I weigh 300 pounds, or I did then, and that meant that each day I used up 4,200 calories. That went on the credit side of my ledger. The debit side used to add up to over 5,000 on most days. If I wanted to lose a pound of fat, I had to cut out 3,500 calories from my debt. That meant, if I cut out 14,000 calories in a week, I'd lose 4 pounds."

"Give me that again."

"Look, spending 4,200 calories a day I use up to 29,400 a week. To lose 4 pounds, I had to limit myself to 15,400 calories a week. Since I know what foods equal what calories, it became a matter of arithmetic. I had been operating in the red—caloriewise—taking in more than I was spending. I had to move over to the black and spend more than I was taking in."

"That's mixed-up bookkeeping!"

"Sure, but this ain't a business. This is a diet. Like the government, I'm happiest when I'm spending. I don't want to balance my books, really. I want to operate at a loss. I call it the *black* because it's the way I want things to come out, but actually it's operating in the *red*."

"Now I know why you sell computers."

"Hey, I'm working out a way of hooking myself into a computer. I'd program it from my little black book and each morning it would go buzz, buzz, click, click and up would pop a card. You are to spend so many calories today. You can eat so much. This for breakfast, this for lunch and this for dinner, click, click!"

"Are you serious?"

"No. The whole point here is to understand your eating habits, why you eat. I know why I eat now. It's a way of assuaging my frustration. I never believed I ate what I did, but my books don't lie. It's all there in black and white.

"Once I understood, I had to recondition myself. I stopped eating on the run, in hotel rooms, at airports or train stations. I ate only at mealtimes and only sitting down at a table. I eat almost all my meals out, and I began to get tough with the waiters. Like, I'd say, 'Take the bread away.' or 'This meat is too fat and I didn't ask for sauce. I want a lean piece. No sauce.' I demanded what I wanted—and I got it."

"I like that. Waiters bully me."

"They like to try it with everyone, but I give them a cold fish-eye and they hop. If they're women, I turn on the charm. I just tell myself, firmly, their job is to serve me, not put me down.

"Another thing, I began to learn that I was very prone to frustration, and it made me eat. Now, when I lose a sale or feel tense, I do something else besides eat."

"What?"

"Well, if my hotel has a gym, I'll work out, or baby myself with a massage, or a sauna, or some steam. Maybe I'll take a hot bath and relax in it, or take a long walk—anything to discharge that tension without eating. It's not so hard once you understand the reason you're eating.

"Another thing, I used to eat like a steam engine. I'd plow through the food one-two-three. Now I eat slowly. If I eat by myself, as I often do, I read a book. That's why I hate dark restaurants. I always ask for a table with the most light, and I prop my book up in front of me and read. I pace myself. So many paragraphs before I take another bite. A page a mouthful goes well, unless you're a speed reader.

"When I'm with a client, it's a little harder, especially if he's a fast eater. I have little tricks, like putting down my fork and knife after each mouthful, and most important—learning to leave something on the plate. But with me, the big thing is slowing down. Now see how long it's taken me to eat his muffin? In the old days, I'd have chomped it down in two bites!"

"But how about your ordering it in the first place?" I asked. "They're very fattening, corn muffins, and after all, this isn't mealtime. We stopped here for a coffee break. Don't tell me your diet lets you eat between meals."

"That's the guilt factor. I've done away with that. In the old days, I'd eat a half pound of halvah and feel guilty about it—

then eat some ice cream to make me feel better about the guilt. Now I eat if I'm hungry. I eat what I crave and then stop. So I fall from grace every few days. No big deal. I just balance my books to include the fall. That way I can enjoy my life after the fall."

He grins as he finishes the last crumbs of the muffin. "I've got it better than Adam and Eve!"

> *Ted's simple technique is a first-rate example of how a little creativity can help you painlessly do something you might otherwise be reluctant to do, such as cutting down on eating. The next time you take on some unexciting task, you, too, might try to tie it in with something you enjoy.*

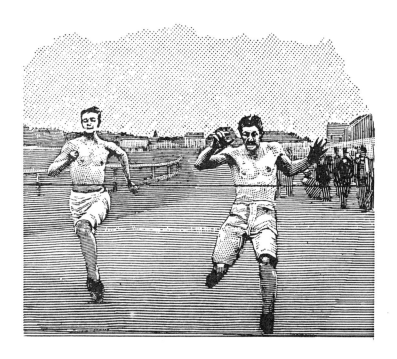

RUNNING HIGH

Almost everyone knows that running is one of the best forms of exercise around. But few know that the right kind of running can give you a sensual high as well.

Carl has been invited for dinner, and Gloria, his first wife, flutters around our house uneasily as dinnertime comes and goes. "I think we'd better eat," she tells us finally. "Carl has a reputation for being late."

"We can wait," I reassure her. "We're having stew, and it's going to keep. Don't worry about it."

·"No, let's eat now," she decides. "You can leave something for Carl." At the table she sighs. "That's really the reason I divorced him."

"Because he's late for dinner?" my wife smiles.

"More than dinner. It's his unreliability. Carl is totally unreliable. Our marriage was a disaster. Our divorce has been fun."

We laugh, realizing that Gloria and Carl have been divorced for thirty years. Gloria married again and was widowed ten years ago. Carl has had four marriages and has been single for eight years. "We've been lovers since his last divorce," Gloria confides, smiling. "It's been wonderful. As long as we don't live together, we get along splendidly." She looks at her watch and sighs. "As long as I don't have to count on him!"

Carl shows up as we're finishing dessert and coffee, and in typical fashion he's covered with sweat, wearing a jogging outfit and sneakers. "Give me five minutes in the bathroom and I'll be a new man," he promises.

We're sitting in the living room with after-dinner brandy when he joins us. "Would you like something to eat?" my wife asks, and he waves the invitation aside. "Some tea would be perfect. No brandy, thanks. I'm fasting today—I fast once a week." His smile dazzles us. "But I didn't want to skip you wonderful people, so I ran over."

"Over" is five miles, and I stare at Carl, a lean, hard sixty and, except for an unruly shock of white hair, looking as if he is in his late forties. Carl is an actor and makes a decent living out of commercials and soaps. Now he leans back and sips his tea. "There is something exciting about running—especially after a day of fasting—that gives you the greatest high in the world. You can keep your uppers and downers, your grass and coke—give me more than a mile of clean running, and I'm stoned!"

"More than a mile?" I ask curiously, marveling at Gloria's calm. She hasn't said one reproving word to Carl. The result of a happy divorce?

"The first mile is always hell, but then all of a sudden it all levels out and you realize you could go on running forever. Something happens to your body, something chemical. Maybe it's just that you produce less lactic acid, or you get rid of the wastes more easily—I don't know, but I'll tell you, if you're a regular runner, you breathe in and use more oxygen than a nonrunner. Maybe that's why, after that first mile, you go into a real high and feel you could keep on forever."

"Do you run often?" I ask.

Carl hits his hard, flat stomach. "You don't get that from walking! I run every day—five to seven miles."

"But you live in the city," I protest. "How do you manage? I know those sidewalks are murder on your feet."

"Oh, I wouldn't run on concrete. You're right about that. They can pound your feet to pieces. I run in the park, usually on the gravel horse path. I walk over there or take a bus, and then I do my five miles. Anyway, I tie up running with trees and lakes. I love to look at nature, green grass or snow-covered fields, while I'm running. It clears out my mind. You know, running also reduces blood pressure. That's a medical fact. My pressure is like a kid of twenty, and my blood cholesterol is way down. The doctors tell me that running increases my coronary circulation and makes me less liable to heart attacks—I've heard that no one who can complete a marathon run ever dies of a heart attack."

"Carl ran in the last city marathon," Gloria says proudly.

"Did you? How did you place?'

Carl laughs. "I came in sixty-seventh out of a hundred, but it was eminently successful for me." He smiles in a self-satisfied way, and Gloria laughs.

"Tell them the whole story," she urges.

Carl doesn't need much urging. "The point is, when I entered I lied about my age."

I nod understandingly. "I guess you'd have to. You must be over sixty and they have to have a cut-off line somewhere."

"No cutoff, but I'm sixty-one and I lied the other way."

"What do you mean?"

"I told them I was seventy-two years old."

I look at him in bewilderment. "But why? Why tell them you're so old? Especially when you're not!"

Enjoying my bewilderment, Carl says, "I even used a little makeup around the eyes to make me look older, though I think I could have gotten away without it."

"But I still don't understand."

"I'll tell you why. Lying like that, I became the oldest man in the marathon—by almost ten years."

A light begins to dawn and I nod. "I think I see."

"But I don't!" my wife says plaintively. "Tell us."

"It's easy. The TV cameras were there to cover the marathon. Running's very big news, but the biggest news was the oldest and the youngest runners. The youngest was a kid of twelve—and I was the oldest. The cameras picked us both up and kept with us. He didn't finish, but I did, and I got me a nice interview on the news that night—a million buck's worth of publicity."

"So that was it!" My wife smiles.

"That was. I got six offers for commercials and two juicy parts in soaps out of that run."

"Plus eleven years," Gloria reminds him.

"Oh well, my birth records were all burned in a city-hall fire down south. This just establishes a different age for Social Security and all that."

A little shocked, I decide to drop that line quickly. "Tell me about your running high."

Carl leans back, sipping his tea. "It *is* a high, you know. One of the greatest pleasures I can get. For one thing, I do it alone, quietly, away from all the craziness of the city and my profession.

"Then, too, I can block all thought out of my mind when I'm running. I just feel the cadence of my feet, the visual input of the scenery, the path, the sky—everything becomes clean and opens up. I guess meditation is the closest thing to it, but along with the high there's this constant expenditure of energy, this strain on my body. It makes me aware of my body, of every muscle, of every impact of my foot against the path. The sort of superawareness is wonderful, exciting and"— he shrugs—"high! There's no other word for it."

"Have you been running long?" My wife asks.

"For twenty years. Would you believe it, I used to be fat and I never did a day's physical work in my life. In fact, I was always cast as the fat man, the comic. I rarely did serious stuff."

Gloria nods. "He was like that when we were married."

"Then I started running, and within a year all the fat had melted off and I began to firm up, all over. I was a different human being, and my health—my God, I haven't been sick one day since then."

"And you run every day!"

"Rain or shine, hot or cold. I run early, especially in the summer to avoid the heat, and to tell the truth, I run for joy, for the sheer joy of it." He looks at his watch. "I'll even run home tonight."

"Not a bit!" Gloria sits up. "Unless you're prepared to carry me. You're driving home with me and staying the night," she adds firmly.

Carl grins. "Okay, you've got a great high school next door to your house."

"What's that got to do with it?" I ask.

"Why it has a half-mile track in back. I'll go."

> *The beauty of running is that you can do it anywhere, anytime, without a heavy investment in equipment. Most communities have parks or high schools with running tracks. You can even run on the sidewalk, but if you do it's advisable to wear running shoes designed for hard surfaces. Start with a few minutes at a time. Soon you'll start looking for new places to run.*

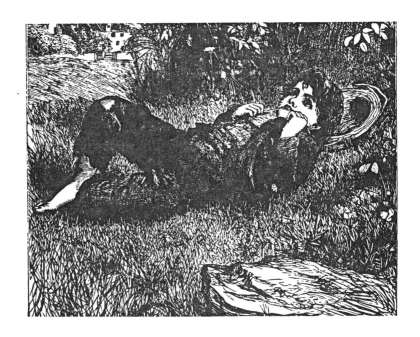

SOLO SENSATIONS

Can you enjoy sex if you're all alone? Here are some ideas.

We were sitting around the living room of Bob's cabin, a rustic, hand-built affair that he had just completed after working on it alone for half a year. The cabin was set in exquisite country in Colorado's San Juan Mountains. It faced across the shores of a small lake to a breathtaking view of mountains to the west.

"You just wouldn't believe the sunsets," Bob told us. "Tonight's was great, but every night seems more beautiful than the last."

Jim shook his head. "I find it incredible that you spent six months here alone putting this up."

Bob nodded. "I learned a lot about building and, you know, a lot about myself. I was lonely in the beginning, but after a while I came to really treasure my loneliness."

"No," Jim said. "What I mean is—well, I'd be bombed out of my skull if I had to give up sex for six months."

There was a moment's awkward silence, and then Bob chuckled. "Who gave it up?"

"But you told us no one came up here, that you didn't see anyone in all that time."

"That's right," Bob said, still smiling.

Judd, who was sixteen, said, "Self-abuse!" with a smart-aleck brightness.

Bob laughed. "It's a joke to you, Judd, and I can see some of you older types looking a little shocked, but I'm twenty-two. My generation grew up without your guilt about masturbation."

Charlotte, in her fifties, laughed nervously. "That word! I feel like Mary Hartman on TV. I want to whisper, 'Don't say it! Don't say it!'"

Bob laughed. "But you see, to me it's a perfectly valid substitute for the real thing. Of course I prefer a woman, but I was isolated here for six months. I had sold my car and everything I had for this land and the building materials. I could hike down to the general store for supplies, but that was it. Don't get me wrong—the sacrifice was well worth it to me. Now I start job-hunting and my life becomes normal again. But for those six months I needed a sexual outlet, and I was damned if I would feel guilty about it."

He frowned. "In fact I found it very beautiful. I'd sit out on the lake side of the cabin watching the sunset, listening to the sounds of the evening and I'd feel a glow of warmth and beauty. I'd feel at one with nature, and nothing seemed more natural than expressing myself sexually."

We were all quiet for a moment. Then Jim said, "It's funny. I had forgotten till now, but three years ago, when Martha went off to Europe for four months on that grant, I was alone and just about ready to climb the walls with good old-fashioned lust. You know, I wouldn't fool around with anyone else. I never have and I hope I never will. I'm very monogamous."

He paused, chewing his lip. "This is an evening for confession and I've had a lot of wine—though this isn't really much of a confession. One night, when I couldn't stand it any longer, I bought a half dozen yellow roses, Martha's favorite flower, and a bottle of really great wine. I put the roses in a vase on the coffee table and lit two candles next to them. I put out all the lights and stood Martha's picture between the candles. Then I dabbed some of her perfume on my chest and put a bit of Mozart on the stereo. I took the phone off the hook, leaned back and—well, there's that ugly word. I masturbated. It wasn't furtive or unhealthy. It was sweet and tender and filled with pleasure and it brought me close to Martha, even though she was half a world away."

"You never told me," Martha said, her eyes moist.

"Well, there it is." Jim sipped his wine.

Judd said, "Hey, man, I feel I ought to make up for that self-abuse crack. We—my generation—we kid about it a lot, but you know, I think we treat it much more casually than you guys. If we need relief, we do it. It's just that, relief. No fuss, no muss."

Charlotte, frowning a little, said, "But I don't think it's healthy."

"It's just as healthy as sex," Judd cut in, "and nowadays no one's about to deny that that's healthy! Physiologically, the same thing happens during masturbation as during sex. To tell you the truth, sometimes it can be a lot better."

"I don't get that," Bob smiles.

"Well, sex depends on your partner. Sex with the wrong person can be too keyed up. Too much may be expected of you, and you may expect too much. Inevitably there's a letdown. When you masturbate, you're in control. You can pace yourself."

"That's a new concept," Bob laughs.

Martha, still a little dewy-eyed, was holding Jim's hand.

"It's a bit different with women," she said slowly. "I guess we're just not as familiar with our genitals. I know there's a big brouhaha nowadays about women learning to masturbate, and I agree that physiologically it's a step toward learning how to respond sexually to a man, but—" she shrugged. "I would do it only if there were no alternative."

Jim nodded. "But I didn't feel I had an alternative."

Smiling at him fondly, Martha said, "I abstained for those four months—but maybe it's easier for a woman."

Sally, Judd's girlfriend, who had been quiet up till now, said, "It's not easier, really. It's a generational thing. Look, it's no sweat to me to masturbate even if I'm without sex for only a few weeks." Turning to Charlotte, she said, "You've been handed too many guilt trips about this. Doing without sex is uncomfortable, and in this crazy society, if we do anything uncomfortable or difficult we all think we're making brownie points. I think if Bob had been, what's the word?—celibate?—for six months, he'd have needed his head cleaned out. My point is, it's no big deal. You go with your feelings."

She shook her head. "As a matter of fact, I'll make a confession. I have a little battery-operated vibrator, and I use that for masturbation, too. Charlotte, don't looked so shocked. Hell, I'm sure when you were my age you never talked like this in mixed company."

Laughing nervously, Charlotte says, "I don't now!"

"Well, it's a good thing we're doing it," Sally insisted. "Men used to have their girlie magazines, and don't tell me they were for anything but sexual arousal leading to guess what. Well, now we women have a few—from *Cosmopolitan* to the raunchier ones—to excite us. The point is, we've got to accept self-love as a way of life. It's always been around. Now we have to face it."

Charlotte sighed. "At least I can accept the phrase self-love without flinching. Oh, intellectually I know you're right, and in all honesty, my life would have been a lot less complicated and a lot easier if I could have gotten rid of my sexual tensions

that easily when I was young. But . . ." She raised her glass
and said wistfully, "I'll drink to the now generation and letting
it all hang out, but Bob, when you do get your car and come
back to civilization—have I got a girl for you!"

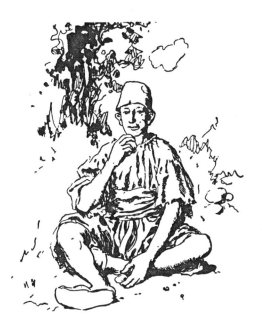

COME TO
YOUR SENSES

Develop your senses and the world will become a much more interesting and beautiful place. Here are some ideas on how to start.

"Do you see that man sitting on the grass?" Nick asks me.

The two of us are having a sandwich on the lawn in the park. Nick has been after me to perfect my awareness, and part of his goal is awareness of my own body. He has insisted that we sit in the lotus position, and the tendons in my legs, unused to such stretching, are protesting painfully. Giving up, I straighten my legs and say, "Yes. I see him, but he's hard to make out because of the grass and bushes behind him. I think it's his gray suit that blends into the background so perfectly."

"Exactly." Nick shakes his head at my physical weakness.

"He fades into the background, but I want you to establish a clear gestalt about that man. Try to become aware of his outline against the background. Stay with his figure. That's the first lesson in awareness: developing your power of concentration."

"I'll try," I promise, and I stare at the seated figure. My problem is, once I have seen him, my attention wanders.

"But you must train yourself to stay with the object, to develop total awareness, to observe every detail. Watch the figure-ground interaction. Life itself, you know, is a continuum of changing interactions."

Looking back at Nick's intense face, I sigh in discouragement. "I just can't do it. Intense boredom sets in!"

"Exactly. Because your senses are jaded, and you need constant stimulation to react. That's why I've brought you out here where the city is far enough away for its stimulation to be weak. I want you to develop an awareness of things. Take this leaf. Look at it and study it. I'll time you. Take five minutes to study it."

Five minutes is an eternity, and I have memorized every spike and vein of the leaf and still have time to spare. I sigh with relief when Nick says, "Enough. You have to practice," he says. "Learn to concentrate. Look at anything—a twig, a blade of grass, your own finger. Concentrate until your awareness takes off."

"But takes off how?"

"There should be a qualitative change in your sense of the object."

I try. That day and afterward, I spend time alone in my room studying a vase, a teacup, a table, looking for that extra touch of awareness; and when I meet Nick again, I think I've found it. "Something has happened," I assure him. "I can't say just what it is, but I think it's an extra depth, an extension of objects out of ordinary space."

"You've hit it!" Nick cries out excitedly, his eyes glowing. "Now you're ready for the next step."

"What's that?"

"Sensory awareness. You know, we understand our environment, the world around us, through our senses—sight, hearing, touch, taste, and smell. I want you to extend all five of those senses until you become aware of a sixth sense."

"How do I do that?"

"You'll start by developing one particular sense, and, paradoxically, the best way to do that is through sensory deprivation, through the temporary loss of that sense."

I am overcome with envy of a man who can use "paradoxically" so casually in coversation. I ask, "How can deprivation increase a sense?"

"Well, let's take the sense of sight. I want you to stay in one room of your house—one you know well, for an hour, blindfolded. Wander around the room. Your other senses will suddenly become stronger and more meaningful."

"I think I see what you're getting at, but will my sense of sight improve?"

"Yes, because afterward you'll look at the room differently."

I follow Nick's suggestion one evening when my wife is off visiting a friend. I blindfold myself carefully and select the living room. At first I walk around tentatively, my arms extended, letting touch and memory guide me. I begin to form an image of the room in my mind, and suddenly another sense awakens—smell. I catch a strong odor of tobacco. That's the ashtray. Can a few cigar ashes give off such a strong smell? A rank, moist odor catches and holds me. I touch the houseplants.

My fingers feel an art nouveau vase. I have always admired its shape, and now my sense of touch explores its etched surface, picking out the cluster of flowers cut into the glass. I begin to be aware of textures in a way I never was before—the leather of the chairs, the velour of the couch, the cold marble of the fireplace. I trace a carved design in the marble, startled that I don't recall ever having seen it.

Now my sense of hearing awakens. There are sounds in the room, the rustling of plant leaves, the creaking of the floor, the noises of the city outside the windows.

When I see Nick again I am genuinely excited. "I think I've felt it, that sixth sense."

"Can you describe it?"

"Not really, but I could feel it. It's not like the other senses. It's more of an awareness. I caught it when I was blindfolded. I was suddenly aware of the room, of everything in it without touching or seeing. If I were a mystic, I'd say it was extrasensory perception."

"I don't think it was," Nick says slowly. "I think it was an amalgam of the other senses. As you increase their sensitivity, they begin to work together and create something startling and new. What about your sense of sight?"

"It was amazing. When I took off the blindfold, I saw things I had never noticed before, things I never realized were there. The designs in my marble fire mantel. I've lived with that fireplace for years, and I never saw the designs before—and they're lovely!"

"So your sight improved through deprivation."

"Paradoxically it did," I say smoothly.

"Good. Now I want you to work on taste."

"Through deprivation?"

"No. Through sensitization. First go on a completely salt-free diet for a day. Then add salt to one food, spaghetti or rice, and savor its taste. Then begin with the spices—rosemary and thyme, oregano and sage, marjoram and sweet basil. Learn to differentiate. Then try a bay leaf. A bay leaf is the test."

"Why?"

"Because it's such a subtle taste. When you've learned to taste bay leaf, then your sense of taste is developed. We'll go on to others."

From taste and a sudden discovery of the subtle differences between the spices, I went on to what Nick called visceral awareness, a sense of my own body and how it worked. I became involved with my pulse; what it was like when I woke up after a nap, or how it felt after a ten-mile run. I discovered its subtle variations; after eating, before bedtime when the weight of the day was still on me, in the company of people I loved and people I couldn't stand.

I began to tense muscles I had never tensed before, to become aware of changes in tension as my urine left my body, after bowel evacuation, after eating—all the physical activities I had always taken for granted.

"Good, good!" Nick assured me. "You're developing. Now I want you to go on to ecological awareness, to get out of yourself and become aware of the world around you. How many wildflowers can you see in the city? In lots, and along streets? Where do you find smooth pebbles in the country? What color is the sky?"

"Blue?"

"And yellow, and green, and pink, and orange—my God, man! There are a multitude of colors in it. And trees—notice the bark of trees, the shape of their leaves, ants and squirrels and birds—ecological awareness, how they all fit together."

"I am a new man," I assure Nick a month later. "My eyes are truly opened to the world around me."

"And your ears? Your taste? All the other senses? Good. You've taken one step toward self-awareness."

Crushed, I ask, "Only one step?"

"Perhaps two. The point is that you understand yourself and you've moved out of yourself. You've become aware of the world around you—or you're beginning to become aware of it. Ecological awareness is one step. We'll go on to an awareness of people, language, culture—a lifetime isn't enough to see and understand!"

"And I always thought I was aware of all that."

"Sure, and you always thought you were aware of your five senses. You never were. Life is a fantastic series of surprises, an opening of door after door."

"Have you ever thought of becoming a guru?"

Nick looks at me with calm, wide eyes. "But I always thought I was!"

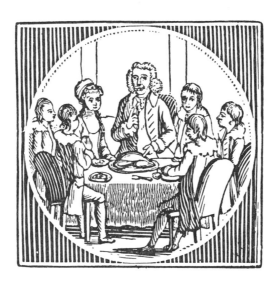

DIETING
IN THE DARK

If you want to go on a diet, but haven't because you don't want to have to tell people you're doing it, here's one way to solve that problem.

It started with an excess of snow on my TV screen. I called Carl, my friendly TV repairman, and he said, "I run into a lot of that. It's the antenna. It sounds as if your booster's shot.

"Normally," Carl confided, "I don't do antenna work, especially those big ones like you got. But things are different now. I'll be over this morning to fix it for you."

I hung up with an awe-inspiring vision of Carl's 250 pounds climbing up my chimney to reach my antenna. If I could get him into a red suit, I'd have the neighborhood thinking it was Christmas. He had that Kris Kringle build!

But when he did show up, I was completely bewildered. Where was the Carl of yesteryear? This was a lean, athletic man, Carl as he might have looked in one of those funny mirrors in an amusement park. "What happened?" I asked.

"Took it off, took it all off!" he said proudly, patting his stomach. "And I've firmed it up with isometrics. I never could stand exercising in front of the family. Makes me feel like a goddamn fool. This isometric stuff is great. When I drive from job to job, I tighten the stomach and relax it. You know that rock music station? I wriggle the belly in time to Elton John. Wow! While I'm working at the bench, I pull in my muscles, tighten them and then relax. I do it while I'm watching TV. I gotta be careful there, though. My wife thought I was developing a twitch.

"But it firmed me up. Here, go ahead, punch me. I'm hard as a rock in my gut. It's a funny thing though. I can't seem to get rid of these 'love handles'—that's what my wife calls them. I know there's no fat left—hell, I'm down to my college weight, but right around my middle here, there's all this flab." He pinched a fold of skin on either side of his body. "How can I get rid of that?"

"You can't," I told him. "No one as fat as you were can. You can take off the fat, but your skin has stretched. How long were you fat?"

"Oh—" He pushed out his lower lip and frowned. "Fifteen, sixteen years. It began the day after I was married. I used to be a skinny kid before that. After the wedding I began to eat, and I haven't stopped since. It piled on slowly in the beginning, or else I was more active then. I used to play sand lot ball, but after the kids came I went way up—and I've stayed up."

"Well, it's a fact of life, the fat can go but the skin stays. Now about this antenna . . ."

With the agility of a mountain goat, or a teen-ager, Carl scaled the ladder to my chimney top and replaced the booster on my antenna. After fixing a few wires with standoffs, he came down and twisted the knobs on my TV. "There, that's a good picture, even on the high-frequency channels."

"Have a cup of coffee with me," I urged, "and tell me about your diet."

Carl accepted the coffee, "Black, with no sugar. Once you
get used to it that way, you can't really stomach cream and
sugar. It's well—like the difference between a boy and a man."

"I don't get that."

"To me, a boy hates raw clams and a man loves them. Same
way with black coffee."

"You mean our palates adjust as we grow older?"

"Whatever. No doughnuts thanks. You know, those doughnuts are one of the richest foods there are—calorically
speaking."

"Would you like a cookie then? Or some crackers and
cheese?"

"No thanks. I don't snack. Coffee or tea between meals,
okay. I'll take an apple while I'm watching TV at night—I
watch a lot of TV, sort of a busman's holiday."

"Why an apple?"

"I guess I could have any fruit, but an apple is satisfying. It's
crunchy and filling. Peaches have less calories, but they're too
soft to fill me up. Pears are okay, if they're real crisp."

"Tell me about your diet."

"Well, it's no big deal. What made me diet? I think it was
one morning when I was showering and I realized how long it
had been since I saw my thing down there. That belly of mine
was in the way.

"That made me think, and I suddenly realized how long it
had been since I'd had sex with my wife—three weeks, and I'm
not even forty years old! I started asking myself, had
something happened to my—what-do-you-call-it—libido? Or
was my wife just disinterested in me? Then I took a long, hard
look at myself in the mirror, stripped, and it was like I really
saw myself, really, for the first time in fifteen years."

Carl was silent for a moment. "You know," he said finally,
"I've tried dieting before because my wife wanted me to, or
the doctor wanted me to, but it never took. This time it did,
and I can tell you—and you can put money on it—I'll never be
fat again."

"What did it?"

"That look at myself, and really seeing myself. I bought a
few calorie tables and decided on an 800-calorie-a-day diet."

"That's pretty hard to stick to."

"Well, I needed to be hard on myself. I didn't want a complicated diet, and I didn't want to shake things up."

"What do you mean, shake things up?"

Carl frowned and scratched his head. "What I mean is, it was my decision, not my wife's or my doctor's this time. I wanted the responsibility—and the pleasure of being thin again all to myself—and I wanted the discomfort, too.

"I usually eat breakfast alone because I leave early to get to the shop before I make my calls. For breakfast I'd have juice, coffee, and toast—the thin sliced white. That makes about 80 calories. For lunch I have a piece of fruit, usually an apple."

"Like your TV snack?"

Carl grinned. "I like apples. They fill me up, and I have a glass of water. I drink a full glass of water with every meal."

"Isn't it rough cutting down so drastically?"

"Oh, for the first day or so, but my motivation was sky-high then. I could have gone through real torture—for a day or two, anyway, and a few days were all I needed to get over the hump."

"What about dinner?"

"I let my wife cook our regular dinner. That's the beauty of this diet. No fuss, no figuring, no turmoil. I was on my own. Look, I dieted right in the middle of the family, and they hardly knew it was happening—at first. What's important is that it didn't upset their routine. The kids and my wife ate the way they usually do."

"But how could you diet eating a regular dinner?"

"Figure it out on a calorie basis. I eat about 140 calories worth of breakfast and lunch. That leaves about 660 for dinner. I cut out little things no one else will notice. Butter, bread, sweets. At first I didn't tell my wife I was dieting. I'd just say, you know, 'The ice cream doesn't agree with me. It upset me the last time I had it.' Or 'My stomach is a little queasy tonight. I'll pass up the pie.' There are a lot of little tricks to keep the family in the dark, at least in the beginning."

"What's the advantage of that?"

He shrugged. "Less hassle. Less guilt if you fail. Anyway, I feel dieting should be a personal matter—but that's just my feeling. I know guys who advertise it to the world, and it works for them. Anyway, you count the calories of an average meal at my house. Chicken and rice with stringbeans and a salad." He takes out a pen and I give him a scrap of paper. "Start with chicken—400 calories for a whole pound. That's more than I can eat. Rice—200 calories for two ounces. You know how much that cooks up to? Stringbeans—20 calories. Salad—40 . . . it's well inside my limit. You know, it's not the meals you sit down to eat that make you fat." He nods at the doughnut I'm chomping. "It's the snacking, the coffee breaks, the refrigerator raids during Johnny Carson—that put it on!"

I agree but point out, "You used a lot of willpower."

"Motivation. That's the secret. You got the motivation? You can diet right in the middle of the family and no one will know—and what's more important, no one will put you off. You tell anyone you're on a diet, and right away they try and push food. Have a doughnut! What a world. Everybody pushes food."

"I'm sorry."

"Hey, I was only kidding." He stood up to go. "Take care of that set now."

I look at the TV with its clear picture of a commercial, a woman thrusting out a plate of spaghetti and murmuring, *"Mangia!"* I know what Carl meant about pushing food—but at least the picture is clear!

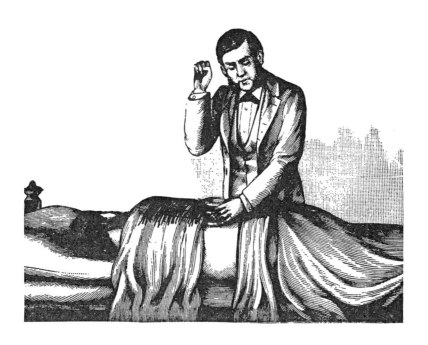

PLEASURE THROUGH PRESSURE

When the pressures of daily life begin to get you down, a different kind of pressure can bring you back up. The Japanese call it shiatzu.

I meet Wendy in the park for a brown-paper-bag picnic on one of the benches, and I'm struck by the glow of health that radiates from her. "You look particularly good today," I tell her, biting into my sandwich. "Is it the fresh air or meeting me?"

"Neither," she laughs. "I've just been pressed awake, and I feel marvelous."

"Pressed awake? That's a new one to me. You'd better explain."

She spreads her hands and gives a little shrug. "I've had acupressure."

"I thought it was acupuncture."

"Well, that's one thing. They stick long, thin needles into you at different pressure points. In *shiatzu*, they don't stick anything in. They just apply pressure to the different points. Like this." She reaches towards me with both hands before I can stop her and presses lightly on either side of my throat. I draw back and Wendy laughs.

"What's *shiatzu*, and what's it got to do with acupressure? I'm completely confused."

"Silly. They're the same thing. Acupressure is just a nickname for *shiatzu*."

"I'll buy that, but what's *shiatzu*?"

"An old Japanese art of pressure therapy. I think it's over four thousand years old. *Shi* means finger and *atzu* means pressure. The idea behind it is that finger pressure on certain vital parts of the body can get rid of your tensions and sort of refresh all your functions."

"Then it's like a massage?"

"Well, not really." Wendy frowns and bites her lip. "You know, it's closer to our chiropractic manipulation—I think. It doesn't *massage* the tissue, it works by pressure at certain key body areas."

"For example?"

"Well, I can't do it to you. It should be done only by someone who's been trained to do it, a professional *shiatzu* therapist trained in Japan who is also a qualified masseur with a license from a state department of health in this country. It's not something to fool around with."

"That's asking a lot."

"*Shiatzu* gives a lot—and if pressure is applied in the wrong way, anywhere on the body, it can do a lot of harm. I tell you, though, my *shiatzu* therapist is teaching me a kind of modified do-it-yourself *shiatzu* to use between sessions."

"How does that work?"

"It's no way as good as the professional therapy, but it can do you some good. It can help you relax. The first thing you have to learn is to regulate your touch. There are three basic *shiatzu* touches: light, medium, and heavy. The light is about 10 pounds, the medium maybe 15, and the heavy is 20."

"What do you mean by pounds?"

"Let's see—the best way I can explain is by pushing against a bathroom scale. Watch the indicator register the number of pounds to your touch. That will teach you control. Let me show you some of the do-it-yourself methods. If you want to get rid of tension and, incidentally, improve the circulation in your face for a better complexion, you use this method."

I tuck the remains of my sandwich into the paper bag and say, "My complexion is pretty good."

"Don't be a smart aleck. Look." She crosses her middle finger over her index and explains, "That increases the pressure on the index finger." Placing both crossed fingers on her neck, one on either side of her windpipe, she says, "Now press here for just three or four seconds, the light pressure. Then you repeat it just below it and work your way down the throat until you are stopped by your clavicle. Got it?"

I nod, crossing my fingers and we both sit facing each other on the park bench, pressing our throats. A startled couple, passing arm in arm, stare at us as they walk on, and I grin at Wendy. "What do you do about feeling self-conscious?"

"Do it alone. Anyway, who cares? It's very healthy. Hey, you always complain about back pain. Try this one. Lean forward and put your hands on your waist with your thumbs to the back, about three inches from your spine. Got it? Now press your thumbs in, hard. This should be a 20-pound pressure. Hold it to the count of three. Wait a few seconds and repeat it—three times altogether.

"Now move your thumbs down three inches on your back and repeat the whole thing. Then move it three inches away from the spine, repeat it and then up to the original level, but now you should be about six inches out from the spine—sort of a big square is covered. See what that does for you."

I follow her instructions uncertainly. It feels fine, but my back didn't hurt to begin with. "I'll try it sometime when I have a real back attack."

"Here's another. Feel around your shoulder with your index finger."

"What am I feeling for?"

"The tenderest spot on your shoulder. When you find it, cross your middle finger over the index and push in hard, 20 pounds of pressure for the count of three. Do that two times on each shoulder."

"What should happen."

"You'll see."

I follow her guide and probe till I find a sensitive area, then push hard. To my surprise, when I stop, there's a sudden feeling of looseness and relaxation in my shoulders. "I don't know if it helped or if it just felt so good to stop."

"You're a doubting Thomas. Now try this one. Cross your fingers and feel behind your head at the base of the skull. There's an indentation there. Push hard again for the count of three. Do it twice and see if you feel anything."

"It feels good."

"Well, try that if you get a headache. It's terrific for the circulation and for easing tension."

Intrigued now, I ask, "Have you any others?"

"Well—I have a routine for my face. First I cross my fingers and press my temples on both sides, twice to the count of three. That's sort of a magical *shiatzu* number. Then, with my thumbs, I press about two inches beyond the corners of my mouth—same count. I press the inner edges of the lower eye ridges, then above the eyes, under the brow bone, close to the nose. I use a light pressure on the inner edges of the eye sockets. I call that my *shiatzu* facial, and it makes my whole face tingle."

I press my eye sockets and cheeks under her directions and try to evaluate the results. "I don't know, Wendy. Maybe my facial muscles are frozen from years of disuse."

"Well, what can I say? It works for me. It's a great way to relax. Try it when you're alone and you'll see."

I followed Wendy's advice bravely in the weeks that followed, and I must admit I found some slight easing of stress and general muscular relaxation when I tried it—more and more as I got into the swing of it. But my real conversion to *shiatzu* came one evening when my wife and I were visiting San Francisco and staying in a Japanese hotel in Japantown.

A friend urged us to try the Japanese baths and specifically mentioned the *shiatzu* therapy given by young Japanese ladies. I recalled Wendy's enthusiasm and decided to take a chance. The baths were fun, a combination of steam heat and hot and cold pools, but ah—the *shiatzu!* I finally understood what Wendy meant.

Stretched out on the massage table, I relaxed as a serious young Japanese woman with almost no command of English probed and pressed up and down the length of my body. Mild pain and discomfort gradually gave way to a physical euphoria that I've rarely experienced.

I showered and dressed and left the baths practically floating on air—and a confirmed convert to *shiatzu!*

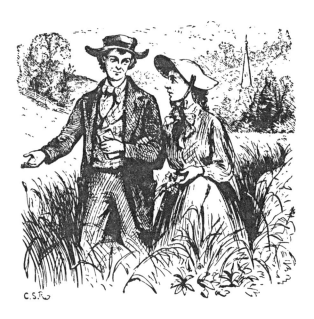

SETTING THE SCENE FOR SEX

In sex, as in almost anything else, surroundings do make a difference—especially if they're new and strange. Take advantage of a change in environment to explore your—and your partner's—sensual potential.

"Have you ever made love in a storm?" Donald asks us.

"I have *loved* up a storm from time to time," Harvey said.

"No, I'm serious. It's the most fantastic sexual turn-on I can think of."

"Those are strong words," I say. "Tell us about it."

Donald sits back and rubs his beard thoughtfully. "It was a few years ago when it first happened. Let's see—I was about twenty-two and I was going with Diane then. She had just rented a studio apartment with a terrace. They called it a penthouse, but it was only one big room. Still, it was on the thirty-second floor of a tremendous city high-rise. The terrace was big and faced west, and she was all excited about growing things on it.

"The apartment had big glass doors opening on the terrace and enormous windows on each side of the doors. It was like a huge glass wall opening into space, and without drapes it gave us the illusion of hanging over the city. Just spectacular!

"Well, we were up there the day her bed arrived—that was all the furniture she had, plus a dozen cardboard cartons—and I had promised to put up bookshelves and do some painting. I remember that it was an afternoon in late June, and there had been an oppressive heat blanketing the city for days. We were both stripped to shorts, and one thing led to another, and eventually to the new bed.

"I had just taken Diane in my arms when she cried out and pointed to the terrace. I looked out and was really awed. For as far as we could see, the sky was a dreadful yellow-brown and the sun a smear of orange. Even as we lay there watching, the sky grew darker and more ominous, and then a huge, jagged sheet of lightning ripped down it and a rumble of thunder came to us.

"Diane shivered and moved back into my arms saying, 'I'm scared, Don.'

"I soothed her, gently stroking her, but I couldn't take my eyes off the sky and the gathering storm. And then the damnedest thing happened to both of us." Donald frowned, his eyes half-closed.

"As the storm grew more intense, our lovemaking grew wilder, too. We seemed to be tuned in to it, caught up in the whole mood of the afternoon. Then the rain came—just furious gusts of it, lightning and thunder—and the more furious the storm, the crazier our sex." He shook his head. "Wow! That afternoon was something for the books. I don't know if Diane was excited by the storm, afraid of it, or a little of both. All I know is how much it affected both of us."

Harvey was smiling as Donald finished. "There's absolutely

no doubt in my mind that the quality of sex, its intensity and pleasure, are all exterior functions."

"What do you mean by that?" I asked.

"I mean that a big part of our sexual enjoyment comes from where we do it, the surroundings. Donald's storm is a case in point. For me, the most exciting sexual experience I ever had was with my wife in our summer house. We were cleaning up early in the season some years ago, and we were together in an upstairs bedroom. It was a hot, humid day, and we were both covered with sweat and half-drugged with the heat. I don't know what turned us on, but we fell on to the bed together, each of us covered with sweat, and somehow—well, it was one of those really exciting, magical moments. But it was the heat that excited both of us, and our sweating bodies—it was as sexual an experience as we've ever had."

"The pleasure of the weather," I told another friend of mine a few days later. "Harvey and Donald were both turned on by the weather. Do you find that strange?"

He shook his head. "No, and I can match their experience, not with heat or storm but the pleasantest sex I ever had was at a beach. It was late at night, and we parked near this stretch of lonely beach and took a blanket down on the sand. We made love on the blanket and everything—the soft night air, the murmur of the surf, the occasional sound of a night-bird calling—it all added up to an exquisite moment—like honey. That's the only way I can describe it."

"No insects biting at you?"

"No. The wind must have been in the right direction."

Smiling, I say, "Now that you mention it, one of the pleasantest sexual experiences my wife and I had was on a summer vacation many years ago. We were staying at a country inn and we took a long walk into the woods one afternoon and started making love there."

"How was it?"

"Fantastic. The leaves of the trees overhead filtered the sunlight down—all pale green and gold. The forest around us was dim and yet alive with color—subdued color really, all muted with green light. There were pine needles all over the ground, and they were as soft as a bed. Our lovemaking had—kind of a holy, religious quality to it, as if it were—somehow sacred."

My friend nodded. "I can understand that. It's atmosphere, the beauty of your forest, of my beach, Harvey's heat and Donald's storm. Exterior forces have a profound effect on sex."

But it's more than atmosphere in the sense of weather or locale, I realize later when I talked to a group of younger, contemporary friends.

"With me," Linda confesses, "it's the back seat of a car in any weather or place."

"That's tacky!" her girlfriend protests. "You're so cramped, and me, I'm always nervous."

"But that's just it," Linda said eagerly. "Being nervous is part of the game. Then sex becomes a little dangerous, more chancy. There's an extra fillip added to it. I like that. I like the discomfort of it, too, the constant feeling we'll be discovered and called down. Sure, it's a hurried, groping kind of sex, but my God, it's exciting! Wow!"

Her friend says slowly, "I like the shower. Now, that's something else again. I remember the first time my boyfriend and I took a shower together. The warm water and the soap—Far out! It turned me on."

Nodding, Linda says, "I've made love in a bathtub."

"Hey, you really dig cramped positions."

"This wasn't cramped. This was in a big, old-fashioned hotel in Europe with enormous bathtubs, and we decided to get in together—sort of conserving water. Well, one thing led to another, and once I thought we'd drown, but we made it, and I tell you true—it was great! Water does some strange things, especially soapy water."

"Speaking of water," another friend cuts in. "I suddenly remember something—have you ever made love in a sailboat?"

"Running in front of the wind?"

"Oh, no, at anchor. We were anchored off Block Island when it happened. It was afternoon, but we were fogged in, so heavy a fog you couldn't even see the length of the boat. I can remember that day so clearly, the motion of the boat, the blankets we had spread on deck, the heavy, heavy fog blanketing us like spun cotton—It was the peculiar quality of the light I remember best, and the motion of the boat as the water rocked it ..." Gil hesitated in sudden bewilderment. "Do you know," he says slowly. "I can recall that day in absolute detail, but for the life of me I can't remember the girl!"

"How typical of a man!" Linda says indignantly.

Gil shakes his head. "No, it was very long ago and I'm sure that girl—she's a woman now—has forgotten all about me, but I'm just as sure she hasn't forgotten that foggy day off Block Island. You see, I believe the sex act is so malleable, so impressionable, that it's as much a product of the environment as it is of the people who make love, and when the environment is different—well, the sex is different, and if the environment is fantastic, or spooky, we remember that and the sex with it—even though we may forget our partners."

"I can't buy that," Linda says. But then her eyes widen a bit. "On the other hand, I have a devil of a time remembering who was with me in that bathtub. I think it was Hal, but it may have been Peter—we were traveling in a group—but I remember the experience!"

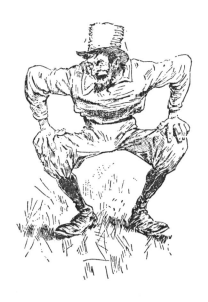

YOU'RE AS YOUNG AS YOU MOVE

No matter how old you are, you never outgrow your need for exercise. All you need is an exercise program that's right for you.

I've promised to pick up my friend Florence and take her to lunch, but when I get to the address she gave me, I find a loft, one flight up, in lower Manhattan. A big sign over the door says *Exercise Class Today*, and I climb the steps, wonderingly. Florence is sixty-four years old. Just what sort of exercise class is she attending?

Inside, I'm completely stunned. A group of golden oldies, men and women from sixty through eighty years of age are lined up in jogging suits, running in place. A trim fifty-year-old man with silver hair blows a whistle and they all stop, breathing heavily. "You can break now," he shouts. "That's all for today."

I catch Florence as she comes out of formation, and I ask, "What the hell is going on here? A geriatric Olympics?"

"Very funny. Come on. I want you to meet Meade, our director." She leads me to the fifty-year-old leader and introduces me. "What goes on here?" I ask curiously. "Aren't all these people too old for exercise?"

A thin, upright man in his eighties with white hair and intense blue eyes snorts angrily. "Believe me, sir. We're just at the age where one needs exercise."

Meade nods agreement. "Sy there had a bad heart condition when he first came to our group. His coronary circulation was so poor that he wasn't even a good candidate for bypass surgery. The doctor he went to told him to go home and sit down."

Sy tosses his head. "Sit down and wait to die was what he meant."

Meade smiles. "Now he can jog a mile without feeling any discomfort, and it's due to our exercise program."

"Tell him about it while I get dressed," Florence says, skipping toward the ladies' locker room.

"It's basically very simple," Meade explains, sitting on the edge of his desk. "This is simply a workshop in fitness for the elderly. You know, you never outgrow your need for exercise, but what happens is that as you grow older, you slow down. You exert yourself less and less. After all, you feel you've earned a rest. Arthritis sets in and you move even less, and then the inevitable heart problems occur."

"But is it safe? Should arthritics and diabetics and heart cases exercise like this?" I ask, nodding around the room.

"Why not? We start gradually."

"You know what I started with?" Sy smiles. "When I first came here, I began by walking across the room and back. After a week, I was walking around the room. Then I began my exercises—damned slow ones, too. Bend to the left, to the right and that was it."

"We build up very slowly," Meade explained. "So slowly it seems almost ridiculous, but we're dealing with fragile bodies, some that have frozen into stiffness. Mrs. Brown! ' he calls out and a slim, erect little woman in her late seventies comes over.

"Yes?"

"Look at Mrs. Brown now. When she came to us she was bent over, cramped. Her back hurt and her joints ached, and she had the beginning of a typical dowager's hump. Some change, huh?"

Little Mrs. Brown smiles. "Posture! I learned to stand erect, to walk erect. Before I ever began exercising, I practiced walking, standing, sitting. For almost a month that was all I did. You don't have to slump and fall in just because you're old. You can get your muscles to tighten up and be as firm as they were when you were thirty or forty. The important thing is consciousness, awareness of your body. You have to force your posture to be good; you have to be aware of your stance every minute of the day."

"You may think we're an old group," Sy put in, "and maybe we are, but every one of us is five or ten years older than we look—and the secret is our bodies, our body language. We speak young—we walk young and stand young!"

"The big trick when you're this age and you decide to start exercising is slowness. You never rush it. Each new movement is done one or two times at first, and then built up, slowly but steadily. You have to go with your body and never exercise beyond the point of tiredness, of discomfort. Never strain yourself. If you get tired, change to something else, use different muscles or else stop altogether till the strain goes away."

"Tell him about posture," Mrs. Brown says. "Tell him what you tell us."

"Why don't you tell him?" Meade smiles.

"Okay!" Her eyes glowing and her back straight, Mrs. Brown says, "You gotta stand tall and proud. Pull in your guts and shove out your hips!"

"And take fifty deep breaths a day," Sy adds, suiting the action to the words.

"But not all at once," Meade cautions. "Do it about five different times, taking ten breaths each time. That's what·Mr. Conrad, who's director of the President's Council on Physical Fitness and Sports, advises. He also advises walking."

"I walk everywhere," Mrs. Brown puts in. "I walk here and I walk home. I walk to the store and everywhere I can."

"Aren't you afraid?" I ask. "I've heard the city streets aren't that safe."

She pushes out her lower lip belligerantly. "Let them try tangling with me. I'm no helpless grandmother!"

"You are a grandmother, though," Meade laughs.

"Oh, sure, but I'm not an old one. I say old's a state of mind."

"What are the advantages of walking?" I ask as Florence, dressed now, joins us.

"It helps the circulation and sends the blood all through the body. That blood nourishes the muscles," Meade explains. "It also helps the heart and helps build up coronary circulation, something older people lose when they neglect exercise."

"Are there any other special precautions for the older exerciser?" I ask.

"Sure. Keep at it," Meade says. "Don't give up if you get tired. Cut back, but don't stop and, let's see—oh, yes. Keep your knees flexed when you exercise. Otherwise you put too much strain on your joints and back."

"And you can lose your balance," Sy adds, flexing his knees and twisting his shoulders."

"Balance is important," Mrs. Brown says. "I often use a chair to hold when I work out at home. I need it, too. At our age, balance isn't too hot."

"A very important thing," Meade says suddenly. "Don't compete. Work at your own speed. Competition is for kids."

Afterward, driving uptown with Florence, I say, "I like your friends. How long have you been going to the group?"

"Months now, and I feel fantastic because of it. And I look better, too, I know. All my friends tell me I do."

"Do you go along with all the instructions Meade gives?"

"Oh, yes. They're important at my age. Like not making

jerky movements, not playing tennis or volleyball or anything competitive. My muscles could tear too easily. And—let's see—I keep a steady pace."

"What do you mean?"

"I don't do all my exercises on weekends, or on one or two nights during the week. I work out a little every day, and I stay away from health clubs."

"Why?"

"The steam rooms and saunas. They're no good for us older folk. Hey, don't get me wrong. I don't baby myself. I do a good two hours of working out, including jogging. I'm pretty good for my age."

I agree. "You are. I hope when I reach my sixties I can start something like that."

"Now, that's where you're all wrong. You should start right now. By the time you're sixty, you should be going strong. You never outgrow your need for exercise—but you're never too young to start."

"Okay. I'll start tomorrow."

"That's more like it!"

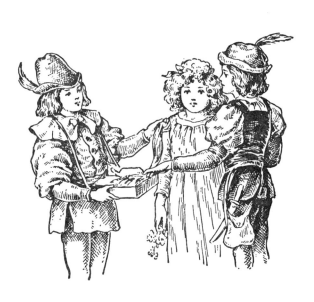

CANDY
IS DANDY

*You probably know candy tastes good, but did you know that
too much of a good thing can sometimes be even better?*

My first experience with gluttony and all its joys came when I
was in the army, still in my early twenties. I was stationed at a
large staging center, and every Saturday night splashy dances
were held in the big rec hall next door to the post library.

On the Saturday night before Valentine's Day, I had a date
with Lynn, a very lovely WAC. We had been going together
for a month while both of us waited for our shipping orders.
On this particular night, she wanted to dance, and I wanted to
read an old potboiler of a mystery I had found.

"Well, read if you want to," she told me, rightfully annoyed as we sat in the library, the music from the dance band bright and enticing. "I'm going to the dance, and here—you might as well keep an eye on this."

This was an enormous heart-shaped box of candy one of the captains had given her. I opened it and asked, "Can I have some?"

"Help yourself."

"You shouldn't date officers," I murmured as she hurried off, and I settled down on one of the library's comfortable couches with my atrocious book and the box of chocolates. The room was empty and dimly lit, and the sound of music from the dance made a pleasant background as I read.

I had a piece of candy and then another and another and another. Slowly, without realizing what was happening, I fell into a delicious state of torpor. In part it was the awful book, and in part the candy. With sugar piling up in my blood-stream, I kept shoveling chocolate into me as I slipped into a half-comatose condition. It was like a dream, and I came out of it with a little shock only when my questing hand found no more chocolate in the box.

Had I really eaten the whole thing? I was shocked out of my "high," and I leafed through the crinkled brown paper wrappers furiously. I had to leave at least one piece for Lynn—but no, every one was gone!

I wrote her an abject apology and left it with the empty box at the front desk. Then I floated back to my barracks, my heart still beating in double time, freaked out on sugar!

I've never forgotten that evening. For one thing, Lynn didn't let me forget it for the few months before we were both shipped out, but over and above her justified complaining, I realized that I had discovered something ecstatic: the joy of unregulated gluttony.

Years later I had another go at that same type of gluttony, and it was just as delightful. It was about a year after I was married and my wife was busy for the evening, so I decided to go to a movie by myself. It was a bad picture she'd never have wasted her time with, but I wanted to see it, and on the way to the theater I passed an old-fashioned candy store.

Memory of the Valentine candy flooded back, and I stopped abruptly and felt through my pockets. I hadn't brought enough money for a box of chocolates, but I did have enough for two pounds of jelly beans. I am, and always have been, a jelly-bean lover. Heaven, at that moment, couldn't contain more than a dreadful movie and all the jelly beans I could eat!

I ate them, too, every last one, spacing them out through the two hours of the movie—something with Bette Davis and a lot of noble sacrifice. It didn't much matter what the movie was because by the end of it I was so high on jelly-bean sugar that I could have floated out of the theater.

"There must be something genetically wrong with me," I confessed to my cousin a few weeks later. "I don't know why I did it any more than I know why I ate Lynn's chocolates, but I loved both of those binges—I loved them!"

My cousin nodded. "I'll go with the genetic factor. Do you see this stomach? Forty extra pounds I've put on since I stopped smoking. Forty!"

"That much? It doesn't look it." My cousin is 6'5", and the extra weight shows up only as a slight thickening around his waist.

"Wait," he said darkly. "This is only the beginning, and I'm powerless to stop it."

"Why? How did you put it on?"

"Halvah. Heavenly, delectable, ecstatic binges with halvah! Do you know what it is?"

"Do I ever!" I thought of halvah, that flaky blend of sesame seeds, almonds, egg white, and honey. Food of the gods! "Yes, I can see a halvah binge—but 40 pounds?"

"I know where to buy it from the barrel. None of that candy-bar stuff for me. I get two pounds of it in one big chunk—it comes in chocolate or vanilla or even pistachio flavor. Sometimes it's marbled. It's so light and it clings to the top of your mouth like peanut butter. What I like to do is get a bag of it and buy a comic book—don't laugh! A real old Superman or Captain Marvel in one of the secondhand stores, and then go into the park and sit down on a bench with the comic book and the halvah and nibble and read till I go into a state of euphoria. Nothing is quite as wonderful!" He pats his stomach. "So I'm 40 pounds overweight. I'll go for 50 or 60—who cares as long as I have my halvah?"

"It's genetic," I decided sadly, my mouth watering for jelly beans as my cousin pours out his secret. But in the years that followed, I was more fortunate than he was. His weight went up as he predicted, but I could control my binges with months between them. And I discovered Turkish delight, gelatinous, light and powdered with sugar. What a food for a glutton!

Over the years I have been done in by divinity—a heavenly candy—by gumdrops, plebian—white chocolate, an anomaly—marzipan—Ah, marzipan! I knew a girl once who had breasts like marzipan, and she drove me mad during my adolescence. I've gotten high on rum balls, on chocolate-covered cherries, on almond macaroons and peanut brittle. On Crackerjacks and those magnificent little chocolate candies with liquor centers.

The highs are all subtly different, and yet similar. I suppose, in the final analysis, it's the destructive sugar coursing through my body and making my heart race dangerously that makes the high, but the taste of the candy has almost as much to do with it.

In later years, with the responsibility of a family and the knowledge of how dangerous sugar can be, my binges are less and less frequent, and eventually, when my children left home for college and marriage I figured that I had finally licked the habit. And then, in a moment of rare betrayal, my wife said, "There's a new store down the street that carries Bassett's ice cream."

"What is Bassett's ice cream?"

"My God! Is it possible you don't know? It's just the best ice cream in the world. It's made in the Reading Terminal in Philadelphia and it's chock full of calories and cholesterol—it's heaven!"

I hurried out with her wistful eyes following me, and I came back with a half-gallon of Irish coffee-flavored ice cream. "We'll never finish it," she said, blushing.

"We'll try," I assured her.

We did, and we did, and in a flood of nostalgia the old sugar high swept over me. "Quick," I told her, "Turn on the TV. Maybe there's an awful old movie or a terrible sitcom."

"Why?"

"I need to round off my high. Don't question it. Just fill my plate again and lean back and eat—oh God, I can't stand it!"

Health researchers discover new dangers in sugar every day—or so it seems to people who love it. I guess I'll just have to put candy in the same category with smoking and drinking: acceptable only in moderation! And only when "paid for" by a commensurate improvement in other health habits.

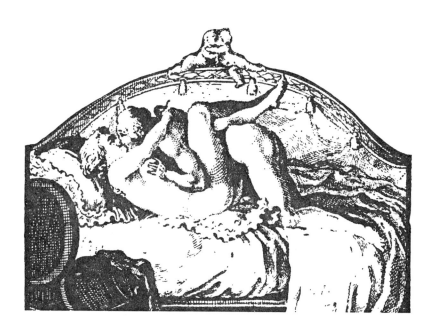

UNBEARABLE DELIGHT INDEFINITELY PROLONGED

What makes the difference between snappy sex and satisfying sex? Here are a few ideas you might want to try.

"What I have wanted to find all my life," Philip says wistfully, "is the secret of unbearable delight indefinitely prolonged." At our blank stares, he goes on. "I read that in a book when I was about ten years old, and I've never been able to forget it. What do you suppose it is?"

Six of us are seated on the back porch of Cora's house up in the mountains. It is dark out and we are sipping wine and eating Cora's remarkable terrine while we listen to the night noises in the woods around us.

"What it is," Hal says bluntly, "is a formula for sexual

intercourse brought to the edge of orgasm and held there for as long as you can."

John, the youngest of us, says, "Wow! Is that possible?"

"According to the Reichians," Alan answers, sipping his wine slowly, "anything is possible in orgasmic terms."

Hal shakes his head. "No. The secret Philip is talking about is much older. I think the Persians first came up with the idea of having sex to the point of orgasm, stopping just short of it till you cooled a bit, then starting again, doing that over and over until you go out of your skull with desire. When the orgasm does come, it's supposed to blow your mind."

Cora laughs. "In my time I've known a lot of men, in the biblical sense, and I will swear that there wasn't one who could hold off like that. Men simply are not equipped to stop short of orgasm more than once or twice—if that much."

"How do you mean, equipped?" John asks.

"I mean psychologically equipped. Start a man on the road to orgasm and nothing will make him stop and reconsider. It's like putting candy in front of a three-month-old baby and telling him not to eat it."

"But the baby doesn't understand."

"And the man does? Come on!"

I say, "I'm sorry you have such a dim view of our sex, Cora, but I can't agree with you. There are men disciplined enough to stop short of orgasm in sex."

"Sure," John says. "Think how many thousands practice withdrawal as a contraceptive measure. That requires exquisite timing and control."

"Well, that's stopping once, but to keep stopping while desire builds up in you . . ."

"I think the original secret must have contained some method for just that, for reaching a plateau and staying there, for withholding orgasmic release indefinitely," Philip suggests.

Laughing, Alice says, "But we women are far ahead of you in that field. We can extend our orgasms almost indefinitely while you poor guys—well, you could use the secret."

"When I was a kid," John says, "and it's funny that I feel free enough to talk of this now—we used to get together, groups of us, and see how often we could masturbate."

"How often?" Cora asks, surprised.

"Well, we'd need a few minutes to recharge, but we'd do it over and over to see what would happen to us. It was weird— the first few times, okay, but then the entire quality of our orgasm changed. It took on a desperate urgency, an exquisite sensation above anything we'd ever experienced. It was a psychological high that was just the greatest!"

Hal shivers. "It sounds like torture."

"We were kids, but in a way I suppose it was torture, but there was that fine line, the sadomasochistic line, where the torture became so exquisite, so exciting—I just can't describe it."

We are all silent for a moment. Then Hal says, "Actually, there are physiological changes that induce changes in your consciousness when you do something like that. There's the fatigue that sets in, of course, but there are inner chemical changes, increases in adrenaline and hormonal secretions that change your body function. I'll tell you one thing: you have to be really dedicated to follow through on something like that. Nature has a way of totally destroying your desire after one or two orgasms."

"Or three or four," John laughs. "We're all different."

"Is any of that like Tantric sex?" Alice asks. "I've heard so many young people talk about it, and I've wondered what it is. Is it your unbearable pleasure indefinitely prolonged?"

"In a sense," John frowns, "you could say so. It's a form of yoga, really. It's supposed to channel the sexual energy, and it uses a very involved series of prayers and chants. It's also heavy on controlled breathing. You have to learn to breathe through each nostril independently."

"That's impossible," Cora protests.

"Not impossible, just difficult. You perform Tantric sex in a special room with candles and incense and bits of food, meat, fish, rice. You bathe first, then the man centers his breathing between his phallus and anus."

Cora giggles. "That I've got to see!"

"I don't think so. It's a very private thing. When the woman comes into the room after her bath, they eat and pray and then get into bed, but in a very stylized manner. The woman takes her clothes off and sits up at the side of the bed. The man repeats certain mantras, admires her, then touches each part of her. I don't know the order because when I tried it I never got that far, but ideally he ends up at her vagina."

"What's next?" Cora asks.

"Well, she raises her legs, brings her knees to her chest, and then he moves to enter her, but once inside he doesn't move. They lie together for about half an hour while the sexual tension builds up. There are all sorts of tricks for preventing orgasm, and in the East, the whole thing takes place without an orgasm. Here, in the impatient West, we're usually not that disciplined. Still, that half hour of not moving is wild, I hear."

"How do you know all that?" Alice asks.

"I once joined a religious commune out in Washington State," John says. "Not Christian religious, but interesting."

"I don't know," Hal says thoughtfully. "The trick would be to keep an erection for that long."

"I think the mantras and exercises help. But to get back to your unbearable delight, Phil," John says thoughtfully. "I think the secret there is in prolonging intercourse."

"But how do you do it?"

"It becomes a matter of technique," John assures him. "Like changing the speed of your movements, or stopping all movement at a crucial point, reciting the multiplication tables, biting your lip till it hurts—oh, I don't know! The point is, if you can hold off long enough the act itself takes over. Your mind and body just drift and you can go on endlessly."

"And when you do let go?"

"Oh, well, it's like fireworks. You plunge the cosmos. There just aren't words to describe it."

"Unbearable delight indefinitely prolonged," Philip whispers. "Someday I have to try it."

"Look!" Cora points to a falling star, a bright streak against the darkening sky, and we all sigh.

"But it's coming down to earth that must be the hardest of all," Hal says softly, and the rest of us are silent in agreement.

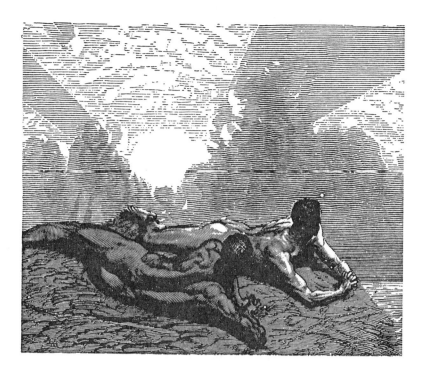

SUN WORSHIP

Hot summer days used to bring me down, until a friend of mine showed me how to master the sun: by giving in to it.

It is one of those exquisitely hot summer days when the whole world seems caught in an inverted brass bowl, and the heat of the sun is almost tangible, something physical that could be cut with a knife. The sky is an unrelenting blue, everywhere except for the area about the sun where it pulses with a hot, golden glow.

I groan and tell Laura, "It's one of those days again, and your cabin hasn't any air conditioning." Then I am ashamed at my own lack of gratitude. Laura has invited me up to her place in the mountains for a weekend away from the city.

"Ah, but the cabin has a lovely redwood deck without a trace of shade and with some comfortable loungers. Come on out and let's work on our tans."

"With a sun like that? I'm neither a mad dog nor an Englishman!"

"You're a saffron-yellow city dweller. Come out in the sun."

"I'll burn horribly and be miserable!"

"Not with my sun lotion. If you're good, I'll do your back."

Later, stretched out in the sun and oiled all over, I slowly become aware of sunlight as an element in itself, a substance as palpable as air or water or earth. It is all around me, pressing down on me, and yet, in an odd way, buoying me up. I can feel it on every part of my skin and it fills me with a languid, lazy, enervating mood. I am suddenly too weak to lift my arms, too weak to even move. I can only submit to the sunlight, let it beat down on me, engulf me and make me a part of itself.

I am on my back, and my closed eyes are staring at the sun. Behind my lids I am suddenly aware of color, a new, exciting kind of color that whirls and breaks and shatters into shards of its complement. It starts as red, and when I press my lids tight, it becomes a velvety brown, darker and darker, but never quite black. And then it explodes in rays of green and red.

"Do you know," I tell Laura softly, "that you can create all kinds of patterns and colors by letting the sun hit your closed eyes?"

"That's phosphene stimulation," she tells me matter-of-factly. "You've heard of seeing stars, the expression?"

"When you're hit on the head?"

"That's it. But just close your eyes anytime and rub them, and you'll see stars. They're subjective images caused by the rods and cones of the eye filtered through the brain. Sometimes, when you take a shower, let the stream of water hit your closed eyes. You'll get some incredible phosphene images. Or just press against your eyeballs and rub. A light pressure gives you a circular, swirling image; a harder pressure gives even crazier images."

"And the sun?"

"What you usually get from sunlight is just a ghost of a pattern—but it's mostly color, swirls of color that shimmer and change. I usually sunbathe with slices of cucumber over my eyes, so I miss out on them."

"Cucumber!"

"Why not? It's cool and refreshing, and I think it helps condition my skin. The only problem is, I miss out on phosphene images, and they're one of the great side pleasures of sunbathing."

"Side pleasures?"

"Well, yes. There's the pleasure of the sun itself, the energy it pours into you, that ecstatic warmth that embraces you and wraps you up in itself."

"Yes," I agree thoughtfully. "I think I know what you mean, now that I've been out here a while. It's almost a palpable thing. You come to feel it all over you, like molten honey."

"You've got it! The other pleasure is the viewing of phosphene images, and when you combine that with the heat of the sunlight, it changes reality. It's as if two of your senses were blocked out—no, changed is more like it. Your sense of touch, when you come to sense the solidity of the sunlight, and your sense of sight, when the phosphene images give you a different dimensional view."

"Are there any other changes?"

"For me, yes. There's the excessive sweating that goes on when I sunbathe. I become dehydrated and even a bit dizzy. I'm fatigued by the sun, and there's a weakness in my arms and legs. Sometimes I stagger when I stand up."

"Is all that good?"

"Yes, It allows me to experience an altered state of consciousness, a condition I never feel in the ordinary run of things. It's a high, a mental and physical high."

"I'll buy that. The sun itself has given me a high."

"Well, I think it's time we both came down from our highs and took a swim."

I sit up reluctantly, and the deck spins around me as the heavy sunshine seems to run off my body, swirling away. For a moment I feel dizzy, and the phosphene images persist, dancing madly in front of me, even though my eyes are open. Then it all sorts itself out, and I shake off the incredible languor that has engulfed me. "I couldn't face a swim!"

"Come along," Laura insists, and leads me off the deck, across the lawn and into the woods. We follow a racing little creek for a few yards until it empties into a wide, still pool in a grassy meadow. It's hardly a hundred feet across and only a few feet deep.

"I couldn't possibly swim in that," I protest. "Two strokes and I'd be across."

"Swim is a euphemism. I want you to float. Floating is almost a part of sunbathing. It completes it, rounds it out. You realize that when you sunbathe at the beach and then float off in the ocean. Now, come on in and abandon yourself!"

I enter the water tentatively, expecting it to be colder than it really is. But the pool is so shallow that the sun has warmed it and I ease myself down with a sigh. Laura is right. It rounds out the sunbathing.

According to Laura, floating is very much like sunbathing. The difference is the water. I consider that self-evident and I tell her so.

"No. What I mean is that in both instances you enter an altered state of consciousness. The sun has a hypnagogic effect. You enter a dream state, and in a sense you float—not physically, but mentally."

Making a note to look up "hypnagogic," I ask, "But mustn't you keep a state of alertness while you're floating?"

"Yes, but your subconscious takes over. In a few minutes you can separate your conscious mind and let an automatic part of your body concentrate on balance. The rest of you goes into a trance. The sun on the water is a different quality than the sun alone or the water alone. You'll see. Float."

I listen to her with only half my mind. The other half is accepting the physical stimuli around me; the sun on my wet skin, the blue of the sky above me, the cool, fragrant breeze from the forest. I float on my back and slowly, gently, I realize that I'm experiencing a new sensual high—something different, so soothing that I am half-asleep, half-awake, and totally relaxed.

I have just started enjoying myself, it seems, when Laura calls out, "It's time now. We'd better get back."

"But I'm so comfortable!"

"That's just it. You need a control when you sunbathe or float. They're both potentially dangerous ways of getting high."

"I don't follow."

"You can forget yourself in the sun and stay out too long, and no matter how much oil you use you'll get burned. In floating, too, you lose track of time."

"And get washed downstream?"

"No, seriously, too much sun or too much water. Neither one is good for you."

"What you're telling me is that I can easily have too much of a good thing."

"That's just what I'm telling you. Towel up and let's go."

The new sunscreens with PABA (para amino benzoic acid) have made it possible for even the "magnolia fair" to stay out and enjoy the sun. But, as with any sensory stimulation, go easy at first. Find your own pace for pleasure.

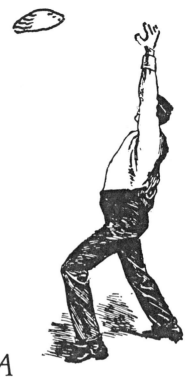

CATCH A
FLYING SAUCER

Here's an activity that's healthy, fun, inexpensive, and beautiful to watch.

"There is nothing," Sanders tells me, "as exquisite as catching and throwing, all in one perfect moment, a Frisbee. It is poetry in motion—the very king of sports."

We are sitting on a park bench watching a group of teenagers sail a Frisbee back and forth. I watch them for a while, then shake my head. "They look like a bunch of clumsy puppies," I tell him. "Half the time they don't even catch the thing. If that's the king of sports, I'll take the queen."

"Well, watch now." He stands up and stretches, all lanky six feet of him. Then he lopes towards the boys. "Hey! Give it here," he yells.

Surprised, the youth stooping to pick up the Frisbee

hesitates, then with a grin sails it toward Sanders. It's a wild throw, I realize, beyond Sanders's reach, and I start to shake my head and smile. Then an amazing thing happens. Sanders's long, attenuated form explodes into action. He races toward the Frisbee, reaching into the air like a ballet dancer doing an extraordinary extension. Suddenly I sit up straight, understanding his remark.

One perfect moment! His leap extends as he catches the Frisbee in midair and completes his movement, coming down to his feet. Then, without a pause, he continues the movement, sweeping around in a circle and, at the end of the turn, he releases the disc and it sails with exquisite grace toward the group of spellbound youngsters.

One of them shakes loose from the spell as the Frisbee floats leisurely toward him. Almost bemused, he reaches out and plucks it from the air. The rest of the group begin to clap in applause as Sanders lopes back to the bench where I'm sitting.

"I am really impressed!" I tell him. "I didn't know you were such an expert."

Before he can answer, the group of youngsters surrounds us. "How'd you do it? What's the trick? Hey, show us!"

Good-naturedly, Sanders gives them a demonstration. "It's all form, form and grace. You have to think of the whole thing as one motion, catching and throwing—one continuous flow of movement. You have to understand how a Frisbee floats—that slow glide toward the end, like a boomerang.

"What you do is move to intercept that glide, and then you move with it. You don't send it back on a different parabola. You catch it on its own orbit and move with that orbit, letting your body complete that ellipse. It's as if you nudged it on its way instead of catching it and then throwing it. You become a part of the Frisbee path. Here, throw it to me again."

Again the Frisbee floats toward him, and again that remarkably graceful catch and throw, and true to his words there's no impact on the path of the floating disc. His hand seems to intercept it and go with it, around and out, giving it a touch of energy as he moves it back—certainly not changing its path. Again, too, it seems to leap into a youngster's waiting hand.

"If you do it right, if your form is perfect, you can aim it anywhere. That's the whole skill of the Frisbee: aiming it just to the waiting hand. Once it starts moving, once you get the right rhythm, it should go back and forth like a feather on the wind, or as if it had its own power source."

Sanders spreads the teen-agers out on the field and moves with them for a while, encouraging, demonstrating and urging them on, scolding them when they miss and complimenting them when they begin to pick up the knack.

When he comes back to the bench to sit with me again, half an hour later, he's still breathing easily, not a bit winded.

"Where did you learn that?" I ask, very impressed. "I never dreamed you had such talent."

"We all hide our lights under bushels," he laughs. "Frisbee tossing is a sadly neglected art. Actually, I just look good because those kids were all so clumsy. Look at them now. Aren't they doing beautifully?"

I shake my head. "You're right. They're much better, more coordinated and graceful, but they can't compare to you. There has to be some sort of story behind this. Come on and tell me."

He laughs and nods. "Okay, there is a story, of course. I started out by demonstrating and selling boomerangs in California, and there's even a story behind that."

"You continue to amaze me."

"I learned how to make them in Australia. I spent five years there after my tour in the army in Vietnam. When I came back to the States it was with an engineering firm—which went out of business pretty quickly. Jobs weren't easy, and while I was collecting unemployment insurance I hung out at the beach, playing with a boomerang for fun and exercise."

"Playing with it?"

"Sure. I'd toss it and when it came back to my hand, I'd catch it. I'd toss and catch, toss and catch. Everything I've said about the Frisbee applies to the boomerang—in spades. You have to really understand the aerodynamics of it to throw it and catch it on its return.

"After a while, I began to collect an audience, and eventually someone offered me five bucks for the boomerang and a lesson. I couldn't resist, broke as I was. So I carved another, and that sold, too, and still another—and within a month I was selling between five and ten a day. It all came just as my unemployment insurance stopped, and I loved doing it. It kept me out in the open air and active. My weight went way down, too."

I look at his lean figure incredulously. "Your weight? Since I've known you you've never been a pound over what you are!"

"Oh, but you didn't know me then. I was way up, maybe twenty pounds overweight. The boomerang business not only kept me in shape, it kept me in food, clothing and shelter. When I got this job and came east I had to give it up—reluctantly, but I had seen the handwriting on the wall."

"What was that?"

"The end of the tourist season. I came east and buckled down to the real world. Then I discovered Frisbees, and it was far out—a whole new dimension of exercise. I'd come out to the park every evening and get up a throw with some of the kids. It's not like a boomerang where you can throw and catch yourself. You need a partner."

"Why didn't you keep at the boomerang game?"

"I tried that for a while, but the same thing happened that happened in California. People kept coming up to me, asking me to sell them the boomerang and teach them how to throw it. I just didn't have the time to become a boomerang maker again. All I wanted was the exercise, so I took up the Frisbee. It's as good as boomerangs and more social."

"Hey!" He jumps up as a wild throw comes near the bench, and he performs his graceful turn and sends the disc sailing back. "Would you like to get into the game?" he asks me.

"Not with you." I shake my head. "You're too much of a pro. I need someone who'll make me look good. I think I'll teach it to my wife."

One of the advantages of this sport is that its fundamentals are so easy to learn. With ten minutes of training, almost anyone can throw a Frisbee. But there is always room for improvement—that's why it's so much fun to practice.

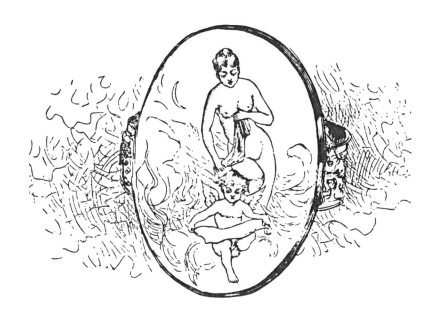

TOUCH
AND GLOW

Ordinary massage has its place. Sometimes, though, the occasion calls for extraordinary massage.

From the moment Jenny and Aaron come into our living room, I am aware of a peculiar tension between them. I don't mean tension in the bad sense—a pulling and tugging—but tension in a positive sense, as if a fine cord connected them at all times, or as if an undercurrent of energy flowed between them. They don't sit together, but each seems to have a peculiar awareness of the other.

We are together to talk about a craft project, the sale of Jenny's exquisitely delicate ceramics. Aaron is acting as her manager, and I have helped by writing some publicity for the new venture. Afterward we have tea and cookies, and I can't resist asking about their relationship.

"You seem so close, so connected. I know you're not married."

"We're lovers," Jenny smiles, "and we live together."

"But it has to be more than that. There's something so right between you."

Aaron laughs and tugs at his handlebar moustache. "It's probably our massage."

"Massage?"

"Yes, Jenny and I are into erotic massage—very much into it—and it's opened up an entirely new dimension in our relationship."

"This you've got to tell me about."

"Both of us love massage," Aaron says easily. "We've been into it for years, with our friends. We give each other massages all the time. In the first place, giving a massage is good exercise. Getting one is a wonderful way to relax, but when two people are in love and massage each other intimately—wow! That is really far out."

"In what way?"

Jenny smiles. "For one thing, it makes sex afterward just great, physically and mentally. I had some friends who had all kinds of sexual problems. I got them into erotic massage, and you know, they learned to trust each other and relax with each other. That was all they needed to get a handle on their sexual problems."

"But even when there are no problems," Aaron adds, "erotic massage is an experience you have to have!"

"Well, what *is* erotic massage?" I ask. "I mean, in what way is it different from ordinary massage?"

"Ordinary massage," Aaron says slowly, "leaves you feeling relaxed. Erotic massage leaves you feeling excited, keyed up, ready for sex."

"Erotic massage," Jenny adds, "focuses on the genitals, but it really excites the entire body. It's sort of as if—you teach the body to feel sexually all over, not just in the genital area."

"How do you do that?"

"You start with an ordinary body massage," Aaron explains. "You cover every part of the body using a light oil. I prefer a vegetable oil because it washes off more easily than baby oil or mineral oil. A scented oil is even better, and a dark room is absolutely necessary.

"You start with the face and work down to the chin, the ears, the neck, and the shoulders. Then you move down to the chest and stomach. If you're a man massaging a woman, there's a special technique for the breasts."

"But doesn't a man always massage a woman in erotic massage?"

Jenny grins. "A woman can massage a man—but you know, two women can give each other erotic massages and so can two men. Not all love is between different sexes."

"I stand corrected. Go on."

"To get back to the breast technique," Aaron continues. "You take a woman's nipple between your two fingers, then open the fingers, massaging away from the nipple, down to the edge of the breast. You do that moving around the breast, like the spokes of a wheel."

"I've found that it turns men on, too," Jenny corrects him.

Aaron nods. "I'll agree, men are very sensitive around the nipples and breast, but that type of stroking is more effective on women. Then you move down to the stomach and upper groin, but you avoid the genitals at this point. The arms come next, and in erotic massage you pay particular attention to the fingers—and to the toes when you do the feet."

"I don't understand that."

Aaron and Jenny grin at each other, then Jenny asks me, almost mischievously, "Aren't the spaces between your toes and fingers particularly sensitive?"

"In what way?"

She laughs. "Well, there are certain parts of the body that simply respond sexually to erotic massage, the toes, the ears, the armpits, the back of the knees—they're almost erogenous zones."

"They *are* erogenous zones," Aaron insists. "Anyway, you finish the arms and legs, and the partner being massaged turns over and you do the back. Up until now, except for the breasts, the massage is exactly like any other body massage. But once you finish the back and start the buttocks, you really get into the erotic area."

"How is that?"

"You run your hand up the back of the legs, right up the buttocks, using two hands on each leg, but you let the inside hand run down between the buttocks, and touch, very lightly, any part of the genital area you can reach."

"But you don't concentrate on the genitals," Jenny warns. "You move up again."

"Anything you do to the buttocks will be exciting," Aaron says. "They're one of the most erotically responsive areas of the body—especially in a man. Jenny runs her fingers around the tip of my coccyx and then works down to the genitals. It drives me wild! Then she brings both hands up from my genitals, up my spine to the back of my neck. It's a great movement."

"Then I concentrate on the buttocks," Jenny says. "I use a lot of pressure and kneading strokes. After that I make Aaron turn over and I massage up from his perineum, just using my forefingers. By then he has an erection—it never fails!" She laughs. "You're blushing."

"Am I really? Put it down to age. Go on."

"The really sexual part starts now," she continues seriously. "I follow along the scrotum and up the sides of the penis and bring my fingers together under the head, then down the other side and around and back to the buttocks. But you have to do it slowly. You have to keep in mind that it's massage, not masturbation."

"That's the important difference," Aaron says seriously. "You must make no attempt to excite your partner to that pitch. Intercourse will come later. Erotic massage is just a way of increasing the sensual and sexual awareness of your body. When I massage Jenny, I use my thumb and forefinger in the vaginal area. I bring my thumbs up from her perineum, around each side to the top of the vagina, and then down again, between the inner and outer lips of the vagina, but I avoid the clitoris. The idea is massage, always massage, not sex."

"But sex after a really good erotic massage is different," Jenny says. "You become so aware of your body and your partner's body. It's as if you learn to feel with every part of your body, and I mean to feel sexually, not just with your genitals."

Aaron laughs. "That's why you seemed to feel that connection between us. It's there all right. We're always aware of each other, tuned into each other's body—I think it's the ultimate trip."

"The *ultimate* body trip," Jenny corrects him and she reaches out to take his hand. I watch, fascinated, almost expecting sparks to fly between them. But they don't need sparks. They are absolutely, completely in tune.

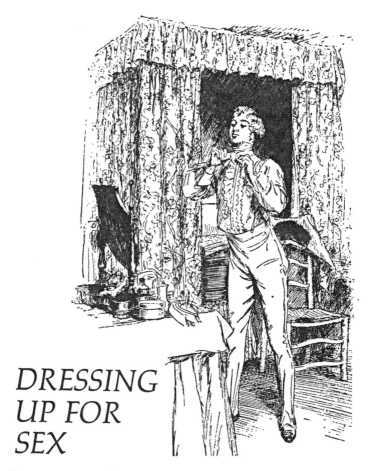

DRESSING UP FOR SEX

If you want to add some pep to a stale relationship, here's an unusual source of inspiration.

"What happened to our marriage—what shook us up about our marriage—was boredom, plain and simple!" Ellen tells me.

"We had been married for just ten years," Ted adds. "In fact, it was on our tenth anniversary that we had a long, serious, heart-to-heart talk that changed our lives."

"In what way?" I ask. Ellen and Ted have invited me for the evening at the suggestion of a mutual friend. "If you're writing about sex," my friend said, "you must meet them. They're a couple who revitalized their entire sex life."

Now, in their very ordinary living room, I look at them curiously. Ellen, a chubby little blond woman pushing forty and Ted, lean, bald and at least five years older. How had they managed to change their life?

"I think I got the idea from that book on femininity—I forget the name—but it was written by some woman who advised wives to make their husbands the center of their universe."

"Did you do that?"

She glances at Ted and giggles. "Some center! No, I thought that was a crock, but in the book she talks about dressing up in see-through nighties and provocative clothes to welcome your husband home from work, and that started me thinking.

"On our anniversary Ted and I had a long, serious talk about our marriage. Ten years, no children and where were we going? It had become a very boring scene. We knew everything there was to know about each other, and in all those years sex had become just a routine, even what nights we had it and when. Wednesday and Saturday nights at eleven. That was it!"

"But you changed?"

"It started because the next day—which was Monday, by the way—I began reading that book and it started me thinking. The author's idea of dressing up hit me. I thought, what if that night, when Ted came home, I met him in some crazy costume? I thought of it at first as just a gag, something to take the sting out of that awful talk we had had the day before, but then I began to wonder—why not something exotic?

"Once I got the idea, I couldn't let it go. I began to worry it the way a dog worries a bone. And then I remembered Ted telling me about an issue of one of those girlie magazines he had bought and how it had really excited him with its illustrations."

"Hey, come on . . ." Ted protests, growing a bit red.

"No, we promised to be honest. Let's tell it the way it was, and maybe it can help someone else. I found the magazine in the den, and there was no question about which illustration he meant. The pages fell right open to it. The girl was not as hefty as I am, but pretty lush, and she was wearing a garter belt, black with a red rose on it, stockings and very high heels. She had been snapped bending over, her back to the camera and peering around at the photographer.

"I really studied that picture, trying to figure out what had turned Ted on, and finally I realized it was the whole thing, the almost naked girl, the garter belt and heels, the pose— everything."

Ellen shakes her head, smiling. "I spent the day getting a duplicate of that garter belt. Thank heaven cloth roses are in. I had to buy one and sew it on a belt. But when I was finished it looked just like the picture. I had the lights low and the room warm and I watched out the window for Ted." She giggles again. "One thing I didn't want—the rare chance he might bring someone home with him. But I saw him come up the walk alone, and I went into my act." She grins at Ted and he laughs.

"How can I tell you what it was like? I opened the door, hung up my coat and called out, 'Ellen?' and she said, 'Come on inside.' I walked in and POW! There she was, bent over, looking back at me, exactly like the picture. I was just stunned and I stood there for a full minute, my throat getting dryer all the time. Then, in a little voice, she whispers, 'What do you say?'"

"What *did* you say?"

"Don't move till I get my pants off! I tell you, that was one hell of an evening. We never got to the bedroom. It all happened there on the living-room carpet. It's a funny thing. I knew it was a charade, an imitation of the picture, but it still excited the hell out of me. The sex we had that night was just sensational."

"And it wasn't even Wednesday!" Ellen laughs. "Ted kept at me after that; 'When are you going to do it again?' But I didn't want to."

"Why not?"

"Well, I was still upset by our talk on our anniversary, and I wanted to be sure sex didn't become the same monotonous thing again, even dressing up for it. I wanted it to be different. I decided that when I did it again, Ted wouldn't know when. It had to be a surprise."

"And then I got this idea," Ted says, his eyes sparkling. "Why couldn't two play at the same game? I began looking for something that would turn Ellen on, some outfit that she associated with sex. We finally found it, if you can believe it, in a gay magazine."

Ellen laughs. "I wonder who those magazines are aimed at! This was a picture of a bald guy in a cowboy hat. You could see he was bald because the hat was pushed way back. I guess the bald head reminded me of Ted. He was wearing Western boots and jeans and his jeans were open, as if he were about to drop them, but you couldn't see anything—I guess that made it sexier. For some reason, that picture excited me so—maybe it was the bald head. I don't know, but Ted got the outfit together and sprang it on me one Sunday when I came home from church. I walked into the house, and there he was! I just . . ." She bites her lip and shakes her head. "My legs were like water. I couldn't even talk and it was as if it wasn't Ted at all, but some exciting stranger—and yet it was Ted!"

"Well, things haven't been the same since," Ted laughs. "Ellen's been after me to repeat that performance, but I'm with her. I'm not about to do the same thing twice. In the meantime we've both been collecting pictures that turn us on, and we spring them on each other. There's no rhyme or reason to when we dress up—and that makes it all the more exciting. We don't know what each other will wear. We get together in the evening and leaf through magazines looking for getups that turn us on sexually. We each collect each other's hang-ups."

"I don't think they're hang-ups," Ellen says thoughtfully. "They're really fantasies. What we do is bring each other's fantasies to life, and sometimes they're pretty far out. Like last week I made Ted put on some of my underwear."

"Hey, come on . . ." Ted protests.

"No, honest. It was strange but it turned us both on, and neither of us knew why."

"I think it was the feel of those feminine fabrics against my skin," Ted says seriously. "They were very sexy."

"And the feminine-masculine mix-up got to me," Ellen nods. "We ought to buy me some cowboy boots and jeans someday."

Looking at her speculatively, Ted says, "Why not?" To me, he adds, "It's the variety, the surprise, the crazy contradictions that get us both—and the fun. All of a sudden, after ten years, sex is fun again. That's worth dressing up for!"

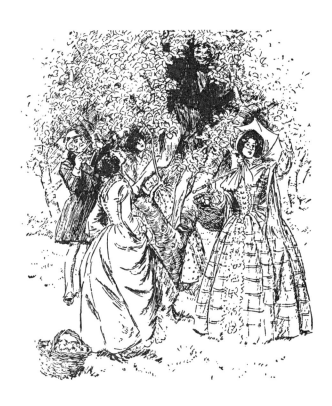

CHILD'S PLAY

An adult who wants to lose weight can choose from a bewildering array of exercise plans and weight-loss programs. Here's a technique that most people never even consider.

"I'm absolutely no good at exercise," Gwen says woefully. "For the life of me, I can't jog regularly or bike or do calisthenics. It all gets so boring, such a drag!"

"Then don't fight it," I tell her. "Relax into sloth. Go with your laziness."

"That's all well and good if you're slim and young enough to burn up all the rich and yummy food you take in. Me, I store it as fat, and without exercise, I'm gradually turning into a shapeless frump. I've seen my roommate give me 'that look,' and I can tell that unless I shape up soon, he'll ship out."

"You *have* got a problem," I agree thoughtfully. We're walking home from an auction on a late afternoon, both of us loaded with packages, and the warm summer weather does nothing to lighten Gwen's mood. "What about a health club?" I suggest.

"Boring, boring, boring!" She shakes her head, and then, as we come abreast of a group of girls playing hopscotch, there's a jingling sound and a chain of keys falls at our feet. One of the girls has made a wild throw.

With an impish grin, Gwen hands me her packages, and, stooping for the keys, calls out, "How about letting me take a turn?"

The girls giggle and nudge each other, then one says, "Go ahead, lady."

Gwen skips over to the series of boxes chalked on the concrete sidewalk, throws the keys, and hops through the complicated pattern, scoops up the keys and hops back. She throws again and gets it perfect, hops, scoops, and throws while I stand watching with a double load of auction "collectibles" and the kids cheer her on.

After fifteen minutes she comes back, breathless and pink-cheeked and grinning like one of the kids. "Here, I'll take those back. Wow—that was fun! I felt as if I were ten years old again."

We walk along and suddenly I say, "You know, I think you've got the answer."

"The answer to what?"

"Your exercise problem."

"You mean . . ." She turns and looks back at the hopscotch game. "That? Hopscotch to take off weight?"

"Look at yourself. You're in a fine sweat and you enjoyed it."

"I certainly did." She chews her lower lip. "And I was good at it, too. They even asked me to stay and play with them. You know, I think you've got the germ of an idea."

"More than a germ—the games kids play, I think you could keep in very good shape that way."

"But it would have to be more than hopscotch. That would get to be a terrible bore."

We pass another group of children jumping rope, one end of the rope tied to the iron part of a stoop, the smallest child turning the other end, and a lineup of girls waiting to jump. One rushes forward and the rest start to chant, "Mary, Mary, she's going to marry Marty, they'll live in Miami, they'll only eat marmalade, they'll name their children Mary, Marty, Manny, Max, Morris, Merry, Melissa . . ."

Gwen turns a glowing face to me, but I shake my head firmly. "First we get these packages back to our apartments!"

I meet Gwen a month later at a friend's house and I'm struck by the difference in her appearance. "You look wonderful," I tell her, guiding her over to a quiet corner. "I can see you've been getting exercise."

"I have, and it's the greatest exercise—I'm having so much fun!" Her eyes sparkle and her whole face seems to glow. She turns slowly for my inspection, smoothing her skirt against her flat stomach. "How do you like the new me?"

"I rather liked the old one, too," I tell her, then add quickly, "But I do like the new one. I like it a lot!"

"Do you know what I've been doing for exercise?"

"Playing hopscotch?"

"Partly. I have a regular game going on at least three times a week, and I'm really a champ and getting better with practice."

"That can't be all."

"Skipping rope, too. Sometimes I do it alone with a small jump rope, and do you know, a half hour of that is absolutely and utterly exhausting! I don't know how kids can go on doing it for hours."

"They're efficient little machines. They turn every bite of food into energy."

"And double Dutch. I'm the double-Dutch expert in the neighborhood. I'm asked into most of the games, and they're glad to have me."

"What other games are you into?"

"Well, the neighborhood kids thought I was some kind of a kook at first—here comes the crazy lady! But after a while they accepted me, especially at jumping rope."

"How come?"

"I guess because I agreed to take double turns at turning. It's for my own good because I just can't keep up with them. Anyway, they've let me play tag with them, and I tell you, that eats up the calories."

I have to laugh at the vision of Gwen playing tag with the girls in the street, but she's small, and in jeans she might blend in. "You're really hooked on this children's games bit."

"More than hooked. It's such a great way to get my exercise. You know my job at the boutique—it doesn't start till noon, and that gives me my mornings free. The streets are full of kids now, at least until school starts. What I'm after, though, are the solitary games, the ones I can do alone when the kids are back in school, games like one-woman jump rope, and single hopscotch."

"Have you found any others?"

"Well, last week my roommate and I took a walk over to the park in the evening. The playground was deserted, but it was still open, so we went in and we began swinging by ourselves. Do you know, swinging takes an awful lot of energy, especially if no one pushes you."

"That's a good single exercise."

"And climbing the monkey bars. Kids scramble up and down them with no effort at all, but it takes some effort for an adult to make it. I can still feel the aches in my leg muscles."

"You may lose your adult privileges if you keep on with this kid stuff. What other games have you discovered?"

"Skipping. That's another heavy exercise, especially if you vary the steps. It becomes something like a dance routine, and it's hard. Let's see—I've stayed away from the games that need mechanical devices."

"Why?"

"I can't see myself scooting along on a skateboard, or a pogo stick. Eventually I'm going to run into a friend or neighbor, and it'll be hard enough explaining simple games. I discarded the idea of roller skates too because I thought they might be as boring as bicycles. But I have found one great solitary sport."

"What's that?"

"Tree climbing. There's a wonderful old cottonwood tree back in the park, and the kids scramble all over it. The other day it was deserted and I said, 'What the hell!' so I heaved myself up to the lowest branch and began to climb. I got so high I could see for miles, the river and the highway. It was so exhilarating, just super. With every foot I climbed back a year into my childhood."

Laughing, I ask, "And your roommate? Are you still afraid he'll ship out?"

Gwen laughs too. "Not anymore. I sent him packing long ago. He thought my games were too undignified, but I've got another, and is he great!"

"In what way?"

"He's taught me to use a Hula Hoop, to fly a kite, and next Sunday he's teaching me a new game called the Australian Pursuit Race."

Fascinated, I ask, "How do you play it?"

"Two can play. You need a big ring or track. Each player starts at opposite ends, and you each run in the same direction. Get the picture? Each one is chasing the other. You run until one catches the other, and he tells me that can really knock you out."

"Do you think you'll catch your roommate?"

"If I don't, he'll catch me. Either way I can't lose."

"I agree with that!"

> If you have children, can you think of a better way to get to know them than to join them in their games? You'll be getting exercise at the same time.

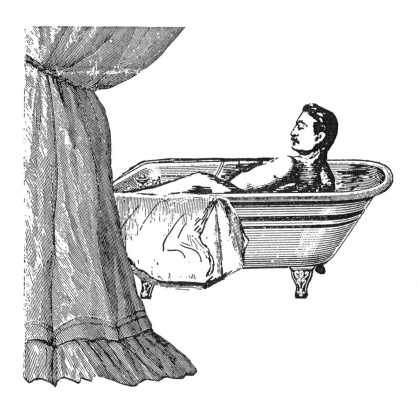

BATHING IN GLORY

When life gets you down, try picking yourself up with an unusual twist on a rather usual habit.

"On those nights—which are increasingly frequent—when I can't sleep, I take my insomniac special," Beatrice says.

Abby looks at Beatrice's sleek, beautifully groomed body with some envy. "I didn't think you ever had trouble coping with anything," she says wistfully. "Let alone sleep!"

"Ah, but my insomniac special is how I cope." There is just the hint of an Italian accent in Beatrice's voice, a remnant of all those years she spent in Milan as beauty consultant for an international cosmetics firm.

"Tell us about it," I say. A group of us are sitting on

Beatrice's back deck after sunset nursing cool drinks and waiting for the summer heat to ease away.

Beatrice stretches lazily. "It's very simple. I run a hot, hot bath, from 100 to 110 degrees, and I just stretch out in it. Fifteen minutes eases every ache out of my body, and it's hypnotic, like a drug. I can barely dry myself afterward and stumble into bed, I'm so sleepy."

"And that's all there is?" Abby sounds disappointed.

"Ah, but that's the skeleton of the treatment. You have to flesh it out. Now, take lighting. For my insomniac special, I turn off all the lights and light just one candle, a scented one. Never a pungent scent. None of the spices, but a soft flower scent. Gardenia is perfect. It's so heavy and cloying, a little hypnotic in itself.

"And music. I have two speakers mounted in my bathroom, fed in from the stereo. I put on something very soft, very sentimental, Montovani maybe. Another thing I'm very careful about is the quality of the water."

"But how can you change that?" I ask.

Beatrice shrugs. "If it's hard, I use a water softener. You know, hard water has all those salts and minerals and they mix with the alkali in the soaps and form hard salts that won't dissolve. It can make a ring around the tub, which is bad enough, but it can also coat your body. You may not see the salt coating, but it keeps you from cleaning your skin properly."

Abby nods. "My skin is dry and sensitive. Is a water softener good for that?"

"Good—but not good enough," Beatrice says positively. "You should use oilated oatmeal in your bath water." Seeing Abby's blank look, she adds kindly, "If you can't get that plain cornstarch will do almost as well."

"Do you use bath oils?" I ask.

"Oh yes, it's a must, but I insist on a dispersible one, one that disperses all through the bath and even penetrates your skin. There's a lovely, smooth feel to the skin after a bath with a good oil—and of course perfume. That's a must, too."

"What I like," Abby says, "is your idea about the candle. It sounds super. I'm just a nut about the visual part of bathing. I have my tub surrounded with plants, and sometimes I'll float a few flowers on the water. I can sink back in the tub and pretend I'm in a jungle pool!"

"Rugs help," Beatrice agrees. "You know, I honestly believe the bathroom is the second most important room in the house."

"Is the bedroom first?" I ask.

"Of course not! The kitchen is first. But you start your day in the bathroom and you can exercise there, and where else can you relax better? To my mind a bathroom can be as alluring and comfortable as the living room—and should be. I like to indulge myself in the bathroom. I have some beautiful prints on the walls, and I always have vases of fresh flowers and plants—they all do well in the moisture. I go all-out with wall coverings and shower curtains and fixtures. I love to pamper myself."

"Pampering is the key," Abby agrees.

"A bathroom is a private place," Beatrice continues seriously, sitting erect in the deck chair. "You want to be alone there. You expect to be alone. It's the one place the rest of the family can't get at you. In my house my bathroom is almost as large as my bedroom—not the guest bathroom, but my private one. Take a look at it later. I have furniture in it, too—a desk and a chair and a chaise—I can relax there."

"You say you keep the water in your bath at over 100 degrees," I ask thoughtfully. "Isn't that too hot for health? Isn't it too enervating?"

"Not for sleep. I want something enervating, soporific, but that's only for my insomniac special. For my regular bath I keep the water at about 98 degrees, the body's temperature. It relaxes nervous and muscular tension without putting you to sleep. I usually follow it with a cool shower or even rub myself down with a towel that's been dipped in cold water and squeezed out."

Abby shivers. "I can't stand cold water!"

"It's very refreshing, and it closes all the pores. In the morning I always take a cool bath—sometimes as cool as 75 degrees. It picks me up for the rest of the day."

"I never bathe in the morning," Abby protests. "I shower. I

save my baths for the evening, after work, especially if I'm going out. I think a bath's a wonderful way to ease out of a day's work. You know, I label my baths in terms of what they do for me."

"What do you mean?" I ask.

"Well, it's a little like Beatrice's insomniac special. I have my calming bath, after a really rough day. I get the water nice and warm but not too hot. I don't know about degrees, so I just feel. I wet a towel and make a neck rest out of it, and sometimes I adjust the water coming in to the water going out through the overflow and I let the incoming water massage my feet. It's kind of heavenly—and I always perfume the water with a few drops of toilet water or a special bath perfume."

"What other baths do you have?" I ask.

"Well, my smell-therapy bath. I usually take that when I've been out shopping or rushing around for some reason or other. I draw a nice, warm bath, put on some relaxing music in the bedroom, that's close enough to hear it if I leave the door open—I think Chopin's études are perfect for a smell bath, then I dump in some lovely scented bath oil or bubble bath and just drift off on a sea of scent."

"I like that sea of scent," I laugh. "Have either of you been writing beauty copy for the magazines?"

"Well, the magazines are not so wrong," Abby says defensively. "There is something therapeutic in lovely scents and oils and bath salts."

"What other baths do you take?"

"I take a spa bath!" Beatrice says brightly. "You can get a mineral bath, packaged just like the ones at famous spas. You empty it into your tub and *voilà!* a spa in your bathroom! Some of them even make the water tingle like champagne. It's fantastic. And afterwards I splash some cologne on my skin. It really brings me alive."

Abby laughs. "I'll confess. I even have toy floating animals near my tub so I can play with them when I bathe."

I shake my head in wonder. "And here I've been showering morning and night simply because it saves so much time."

"But that's where you're wrong," Beatrice protests. "Save

time for what. It's rush, rush, rush—to get where? You're like the swallow who bartered his soul for speed and forgot he way to the south."

"I like that."

"But seriously, you must learn to relax. Why do you think we women outlive you men?"

"I think it's genetics. Right?"

"Nonsense. It's because we've learned to slow down. We take care of ourselves. We pamper our bodies and we live longer."

"All that from a bath!" I marvel. "I think I'll try one tonight. But you know, I never could relax for any time in a tub without something to occupy me. I'll take a book in with me."

"Of course!" Abby sits up with a happy expression. "You've discovered another—the literary bath!"

> *You might also want to consider the culinary bath (breakfast in bath), the telephonic bath (use a speakerphone so you won't get a shock), or even the productive bath (bring in a pad of paper and write letters).*

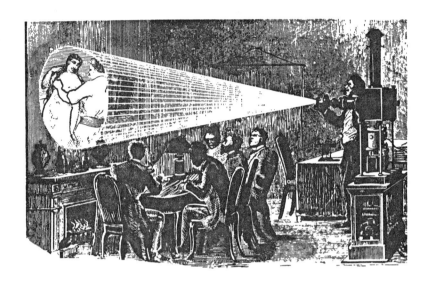

MY LOVE IS
BLUE (MOVIES)

"Blue movies"—also known as porno films—have a seedy reputation that may be entirely warranted. Here's how a friend opened my mind to a new attitude toward them.

"Have you ever gone to a porno flick?" Josh asks.

The question seems threatening. I never have, but if I admit it, I'll be considered old-fashioned, square. If I lie and say yes, I'll have to discuss something I know nothing about. I stall and say, "Well—not quite."

"Not quite?" Josh professes bewilderment. "Does that mean yes or no?"

My friend Ellen, who's been enjoying my embarrassment, says, "It sounds like a reluctant no."

"Well, I have seen some X-rated movies. I saw *Last Tango in Paris.*"

Josh waves this aside. "That's soft-core. I mean a real, hard-core pornographic flick."

I shake my head. "I guess the answer is no."

"Well, you have really missed out on something. A really good hard-core porno film is the living end in excitement and stimulation."

"I'll bet."

"I mean that seriously. I'm convinced they're becoming an art form."

"Ah, come on," I protest. "How can you say that? They're produced by sleazy outfits, backed by gangster money and aimed at the lowest common denominator in audiences!"

"I object to that," Josh says. "First you tell me you've never seen one, and now here you are ready to pass judgment on the men who make them and the men who see them."

"I've read about them," I say stiffly, recognizing the weakness of my position.

"But you haven't seen one. That's the point, and I've seen dozens. I find that they turn me on, and I refuse to believe that I'm the lowest common denominator in audiences."

Intrigued, I ask, "But what do you like about them? Specifically, what do you like?"

Josh sits up and frowns. "Now let me take that question seriously. First, the turn-on. I get physically excited. My body responds. I even think my temperature rises. I get the same physiological reaction I get when I become interested in a sexy girl, when I neck with her."

"What do you mean by physically excited?"

"Oh, come on. You know what I mean. I get an erection. I respond on a sexual level."

"But seriously, Josh," I protest. "What's the fun in that if you're not able to follow through and satisfy yourself—or do you?"

"No, I don't. Oh, some people do, but I don't. But for that matter, I've spent nights with girls making love without having intercourse—and it was enjoyable. I got a charge out of it. I had the same physical reaction but I didn't, for one reason or another—usually the girl's wishes—follow through—any more than I do in a porno movie."

"But don't you get frustrated?"

"Life, if you examine it closely, is made up of frustrations. Sure, I get frustrated. I get frustrated if I take an attractive woman out and can't score, but the frustration doesn't destroy the fun I get from taking her out."

"I can go along with that," Ellen says thoughtfully. "Women understand that kind of frustration."

"More than men?"

"Sure. We're raised to hold back sexually. Men are raised to try to break down our resistance. Just because we don't go all the way sexually doesn't mean we don't enjoy the struggle."

"There's another thing," Josh says. "I enjoy watching naked ladies in the sexual act. It improves my fantasy life."

"Is that good?"

"Sure it is. There's a feedback in operation. My sexual fantasy life influences my real sexual life. If I have sex the evening after, or even a few days after, I've seen a porno flick, it becomes much more intense, much more exciting—and, best of all, if I see a porno flick with a woman and then have sex with her afterwards, it works for both of us. We're both turned on. Somehow sex becomes better."

"Better in what way?" I ask. "You mean perform better, you copy what you see in the movie?"

"No, not at all. I don't need porno movies to give me ideas. What happens is psychological. There's a change in intensity. Sex becomes more intense; my reactions are more intense. You know, I once took a woman I had been dating to a porno movie. Sex had been all right between us—or at least I thought it had—but during that film we both became very aroused and sex afterward was fantastic—much richer and fuller."

"But from everything I've heard," Ellen says, "those films haven't any real plot, no real story. Is it just sex?"

"Plot and story? No, not really, though some porno movies try to have them. The best you can say is that some have situations that lead up to the sex, and I'll admit that they're all poorly made with atrocious acting, but you know, I find them more true-to-life than most of the romantic crap that's ground out in the legitimate films."

"Oh, come on! True to life? What kind of a life do you lead?"

Josh laughs. "You're a staid married man. Me, I'm a young swinger. You know, I've even rented porno movies and shown them in my own home."

"To whom?" I had a vision of a social evening with an announcement to my guests, "And now for some unusual entertainment . . ." "I find that a little wild!" I tell Josh.

"Wild's the word. I once showed a porno movie to a woman I was trying to get into the sack—don't laugh. It worked! I've shown them at parties, too."

"What happened?"

For the first time Josh looks embarrassed. "It turned into an orgy."

"I think what we have here is a generation gap . . ." I begin, but Josh shakes his head.

"I know plenty of couples your age who go to all the porno movies, and you know—a lot of them claim it helps their marriage."

"Sort of charges up their batteries?"

"Let me tell you, on a cold morning your car isn't the only thing that needs a charge."

"It's more than a generation gap," Ellen decides. "What we have here is a clash of life-styles—and you know, I think I'm in the middle. I've never seen a porno film, but someday I think I might."

"I'll take you," Josh offers quickly.

Looking at him thoughtfully, Ellen shakes her head. "Uh-uh. After this little talk, your motives are suspect. I'll go with a friend—a platonic friend. I'm not yet ready for your sexual revolution."

Sighing, I say, "Well, if I've missed the sexual revolution, at least my wife and I missed it together."

Some sex therapists have advised couples with sexual problems to see "adult" films together. Those who dislike the idea of being seen at a XXX-rated feature may prefer to rent the films and watch them in the privacy of their homes.

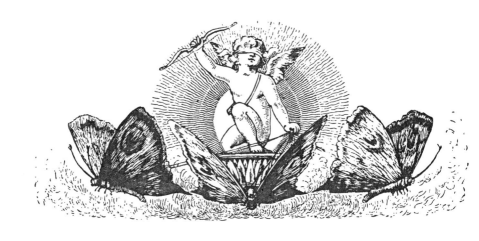

THE LOVERS' DIET

Two can diet as easily as one, if they know how to do it. Here's a technique that doesn't leave room for excuses.

"I've heard that inside every fat girl there's a thin girl struggling to get out," I tell my ex-fat friend Amber.

She smooths her dress down around her ample, but now not too generous hips, and then reaches across to take Frank's hand. "No way. The truth is, inside every fat girl there's a fatter one trying to get out. That's the big trouble. No matter how much weight I take off—and I've taken off over twenty pounds in the last six months—I still see myself as a fat girl. I know I'm a fat girl, and I'll always be one. Fat is a state of mind."

Frank looks at her with fond tolerance. "What Amber means is self-image. We all have images of ourselves, and reality often doesn't coincide with that image."

Amber takes her hand away with a little frown. "I don't like to be told what I mean."

"What do you mean?" I ask.

"Just what Frank said. That's the way I see myself—fat! No matter how much I lose. Now I'm down to 150 pounds, and I'm five foot nine and big-boned. I can't get much below this, but do I look in the mirror and see a well-built woman? Wrong. I see a fatty. I've always seen a fatty and I always will. I think that's why dieting is so hard. I lose the weight, but I don't see any difference."

"But I see it," Frank protests. "You have to learn to see through my eyes."

Frowning again, Amber says, "I want to see with *my* own eyes. I want to be my own woman. I love you, Frank, but I don't want you to devour me!"

Grinning, Frank says, "It always gets back to eating with us. You know, we met at Weight Watchers."

I'm surprised at this. At twenty-seven, Frank has a solid build, but his stomach is flat and his arms, below his T-shirt, are well muscled. "You don't look as if you ever needed Weight Watchers."

"Oh, but I did. I still do. I can put on a pound or two just by browsing through a cookbook. You know, out here in Salt Lake City we have a bakery that uses real butter. Well, I can walk past their doors and put on weight by osmosis."

"To tell you the truth," Amber says ruefully, "we were both dropouts from Weight Watchers. In the four months we attended we each gained five pounds."

"It was all that talk about food, the constant dwelling on it," Frank says. "Weighing our food, planning our menus, becoming so goddamn involved with eating! It made me hungrier than ever, and I ate more than ever."

"But I've known so many people who've lost weight at Weight Watchers," I protest.

"Oh, yes," Amber puts in. "That's very true. My girlfriend

Jenny is taking it off steadily, and she's a regular attender. But for us—well, once we met and began going together, we moved in with each other and what Frank says is true. All that obsession with food! If we were feeling low or lonely, we'd turn to the refrigerator. Do you know, I'd get up from watching a TV show and walk into the kitchen, open the refrigerator, and just look at it. It was a place to go when I was restless or bored."

"But you did take off the weight."

"We both did," Amber says, smiling at Frank, "and it was very simple. I think you could call it 'The Lovers' Diet.'"

"What we realized," Frank explained, "is that we were involved with food, sure, but we were also involved with each other—to an obsessive degree."

"I wouldn't call it obsessive," Amber says quickly. "We were in love. Don't be afraid to say it, Frank."

"I'm not afraid," he grins at her fondly. "I'll shout it from the goddamn rooftops! We were obsessively in love!"

"Oh, Frank!"

"All right—but the point is," he explains to me seriously, "the answer to it hit us one afternoon when we met during lunch hour and went into a restaurant to eat and talk. We both ordered sandwiches, but they ran out of the bologna I ordered and just brought Amber's bacon, lettuce, and tomato. It was crowded, and I couldn't get the waitress's eye and finally Amber said, 'Here. Have half of mine.' I did, and you know, we were both satisfied. The waitress never brought me my order, and afterward I began to think, maybe the problem wasn't so much in what we ate—this type of food or that, so much fish to so much meat to so much fruit and salad, the way Weight Watchers stress—as it was in the *amount* we ate."

"Doesn't everyone know that?"

"Maybe, but sometimes you don't know it consciously, or unconsciously. Which is it? Look, it's like what we said about self-image. I look in a mirror and I see I'm not fat, but inside me there's this fat girl pointing a finger and yelling, 'Hey, fatso! Take it off!' It's that kind of knowing."

"We were so involved in what we should eat that we forgot

about how much we should eat," Frank explains slowly. "And we were bombarded with diets that said, 'Eat as much as you want and take it off.' The all-fat diet or the carbohydrate diet— this sharing, splitting that BLT sandwich, well, it began what Amber and I call our Lovers' Diet. We split things. Sometimes we'll want dessert. We don't fight it too hard. We order one and split it. We split our sandwiches when we eat out, or if it's at night, we split our dinner."

"How do you do that?"

"I'll order a full dinner and Amber will order an extra plate. So they charge us a buck or two extra. We save on the price of the single meal—and on that little extra weight we don't put on."

"Aren't you hungry afterward?"

"Oddly enough we're not as hungry as we used to be on those involved diets. And we work out little tricks."

"Yes," Amber puts in, "Like the 'please, no rolls or bread' bit."

"What's that?"

"Before we order, we say, 'Please, no bread.' That removes temptation. Another thing. At the beginning of the meal, when the waiter brings the main course, we make a big noise about how we must have a doggie bag."

"Right at the beginning," Frank nods. "That locks us in. Then we have to leave enough to put in the bag or we'll look silly when the waiter or waitress comes round with it."

"What other lovers' tricks do you use?"

Amber gives Frank a sly look and then says, "We feed each other."

"Tell me about that."

Trying not to look silly, Frank says, "We'll do it when we eat at home. We set up the whole schtick, candlelight, beautiful linen on the table, Amber's silver she inherited from her grandmother—soft background music . . ."

"Debussy," Amber says, cuddling up to Frank.

"Then we feed each other. It slows things up enormously."

"Sometimes Frank will nibble food from my lips," Amber says softly. "What starts as nibbles become kisses." She shrugs. "That slows it all up even more. We rarely get to the dessert."

"You *are* the dessert," Frank declares, lifting her hand and kissing her fingers.

Amber giggles and I get up to go. "I think I'll leave you two to your dessert."

But they're too absorbed in the last course to hear me.

When you're planning a diet, the first problem you have to solve is commitment: how do you make sure you'll stick with it? The ideas this couple just described might help you come up with some of your own.

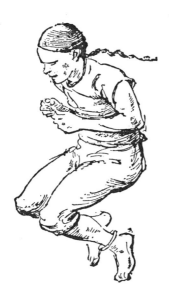

TEN MINUTES AGAINST TENSION

An ancient Chinese art can help you escape the tensions of modern life. You can use this technique almost anywhere, in ten minutes or less.

It was a long drive from San Francisco to Chico to visit Jack's mother, and after two hours I stopped the car to give us both a chance to stretch. I did a few deep bends, touching my toes to loosen up, but Jack, to my bewilderment, went into a series of graceful movements for all the world like a ballet dancer in slow motion.

"What on earth are you doing?" I asked.

Smiling serenely, he said, *"T'ai Chi."* Then he continued, bending his knees, rocking forward on one leg then back on another, all the while moving his hands, palm up, palm down, elbows bent, elbows straight.

I watched, halfway between laughter and fascination. Later, back in the car, I asked him, "What was that all about?"

"Well, it loosened me up, took all the tension of driving out of me."

"*T'ai Chi*—sounds like a game of Chinese checkers. What is it?" I asked curiously.

"It's nothing new, you know. In fact it's been around for literally thousands of years."

"Not around me!"

"The full name is *T'ai Chi Chuan,* and basically it consists of the fundamental movements that all the martial arts are based on."

"Now the martial arts I've heard of. Jujitsu and karate—I even used to be a Bruce Lee fan, but I remember the martial being very fast. Hup, hup, and a quick deck with the back of the hand—or maybe a foot. I'm a James Bond fan, too."

"Well, speed up *T'ai Chi* and you get your hup, hup, and chop. Do you know, there are over a hundred different movements in *T'ai Chi.* I know only six of them. I run through them about ten times each morning when I get up."

I looked at him curiously, then back at the road. "What do they do for you?"

"Well"—he hesitated—"If I do them, I feel terrific for the rest of the day, relaxed and—I don't know, up. Yeah, that's it! I feel up."

"Always?"

Bruce shrugged. "Of course it depends on how I feel before I start."

I laughed at that. "Seriously, aren't these exercises you were doing simply bending and stretching?"

He shook his head. "They may look easy, but you know, it took me weeks to learn them. They require an immense amount of coordination and balance. They exercise every muscle and bone in your body."

"I find that hard to believe. That simple routine you did?"

"Yes. You see, it puts your weight on different balance points. The hard part is learning to do it with a flowing motion. Do you know, the ancient Chinese used to do it for an hour every morning. I do it for ten minutes and it changes my entire outlook. Can you imagine what it did for the Chinese?"

"Before Mao?"

"Now, too. Watch some of the newsreels. Their calisthenics are based on *T'ai Chi*—I think that's why Chinese often live longer than Western people."

"Because of *T'ai Chi?*"

"In part, but remember, *T'ai Chi* is more than physical. You cleanse your mind while doing it by concentrating on the movements alone. It's really a form of meditation through body movement."

"I don't think, therefore I am not."

"Just stop resisting." Jack lifted his hands, palms out. "Try to be open about this. You know, we all have lines of energy flowing through our body."

"Actually I didn't know."

"*T'ai Chi* realigns those lines of energy and takes in the subtle vibrations of the cosmos."

"Come on—"

"No, listen. Like all machines, humans absorb vibrations and respond to them."

"I don't think of myself as a machine." I twisted the wheel and the car responded. "Now that's a machine."

Jack sighed and was silent for a while, then took a new tack. "The idea behind much of *T'ai Chi* is proper breathing. Breathing is our connection with the infinite . . ." He paused at the look on my face, and then said, "All right. I'll keep it on a physical level."

"That's the level I live on."

"*T'ai Chi* teaches you to breathe deeply and slowly, from the stomach. You breathe in slowly and exhale slowly. That kind of breathing relaxes me. It loosens my entire body, frees my movements."

"Do you enjoy it? I mean doing it, not the results."

"Oh, yes," he said quickly, and then hesitated. "At least when I'm feeling good. Of course, it's not a panacea. Still, when I have bad feelings, it cuts them down."

"How?"

"By stopping my anxieties."

"Really?"

"Well, sometimes. You see, while you're doing it, you get into a rhythm that calms you."

"But aren't the anxieties still there? What if you're anxious about real things?"

"Hey, it's not a miracle. Real problems have to be solved. *T'ai Chi* cuts down your excessive worrying about real things."

"Can you do *T'ai Chi* during the day, when you feel overwhelmed?"

"You just saw me do it to relieve tension."

"But that was physical tension from being cramped in the car."

"It helps that, too—and the emotional tension of your driving."

"Thanks!" I accelerated to pass a truck and swung in ahead of it. Glancing sideways, I saw that Jack had his eyes closed and his hands bent in a *T'ai Chi* position.

Catching my glance, he smiled. "That's the waterfall position."

"For passing autos?"

"For reckless driving. It may not help, but it takes my mind off it. Don't mind me. Drive on."

Many cities have T'ai Chi studios. Look in the Yellow Pages under "Judo Instruction," but remember that while T'ai Chi and judo are both "martial arts," their uses are entirely different. You might also visit a well-stocked bookstore, since quite a few good books on T'ai Chi are now available.

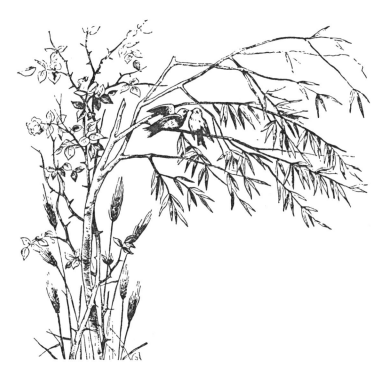

SPICE UP
YOUR SEX LIFE

You've probably heard that dieting can improve an overweight person's sex life. One friend of mine discovered a diet that'll double the fun.

"I cannot agree with those two," Sheldon told me, annoyance in his voice, after reading Frank and Amber's Lovers' Diet.

"I don't think they were completely serious," I tell him placatingly. We've met during the lunch hour in a small city park, and Sheldon, a rangy six-footer, leans back on the park bench, his legs thrust out.

"Love is something we've got to take seriously," he frowns. "Are you, or Amber or Frank aware that there is a definite aphrodisiacal potential in certain spices? Do you know that starting any diet with a one-day fast of herbal tea laxative—to clean your system—plus fruit juice can increase your sexual potential?"

"I didn't know that," I say, smiling. "I'm not even sure that it's true."

"You can believe me," Sheldon nods. "I've been that route. The secret of the real sexual diet is nature. You've got to get back to nature, to the way nature meant us to eat."

"I don't really think of nature as a sentient force," I say seriously.

"Well, man it is! Whatever you may think, it is. But in any case, it's natural foods that get the juices flowing and raise a lot of things—including your body heat."

"Now give me an example," I protest. "I can't take all this vague talk of natural foods. Aren't all foods natural?"

Sheldon sits up straighter. "Maybe I was being vague. What I'm talking about is a real vegetarian diet with a strong accent on herbs. You see, herbs can be aphrodisiac. That's a well-known fact."

"Not to me it isn't. What herbs?"

"Let's take sarsaparilla tea. That contains the male hormone, and turtle soup—that rejuvenates men's glands, and paprika. That's a sexy spice. Or curry, rosemary, cumin, thyme . . .'"

"Now, hold on. I don't believe for one moment that sarsaparilla, which comes from the roots of a plant, can contain the male hormone. And turtle soup? What kind of a vegetarian diet is that? And how does it figure to be a spice?"

"Well—a turtle's a reptile. What I say is, you have to clean your system of meats. It doesn't have to be totally vegetarian. You can eat eggs because the cholesterol in eggs is a base for the male hormones."

"I'll go along with that much."

"And certain spices, if you want me to be very technical, have a gently irritating tingling effect on the genital tract. That's an aphrodisiac action."

"What spices?"

"Curry, cayenne pepper—and there's an African drug that you can buy in some health food shops called yohimbin. It dilates the blood vessels in the genitals. Oh, it may make you a little weak because it also lowers your blood pressure, but it's effective."

"It sounds like witchcraft."

"Well, maybe it is. Maybe some witches know a sight more than modern doctors. You know why Porfirio Rubirosa was such a great lover?"

"Tell me."

"He took a certain elixir, recommended by a witch-woman, regularly. It's called Pega Palo Fortidorn, and it comes from the Dominican Republic. They're closer to the soil there. They know about those things—oh, not scientifically, but empirically."

"And you mix these herbs with a vegetable diet?"

"Right. To lose weight and gain sexual prowess."

"Tell me about the diet."

Sheldon considers. "It's not so complicated. You can stay on it as long as you want—you won't miss any important nourishment, but if you want to, you can take vitamins with it."

"I thought it was natural."

"Sure. So take natural vitamins. Me, when I go on the diet, I take brewer's yeast and a tablespoon of blackstrap molasses diluted in a little cider vinegar each day. That gives me all the vitamins, minerals, lecithin, and iron I need."

"And the diet?"

"Let's see. Breakfast is always the same. You have two thin slices of toast with a little butter and honey on it, and you drink ginseng tea. That's if you want to lose weight. If you're just dieting for the sexual hell of it, you can add berries and wheat germ, or dried fruits and nuts, or oatmeal. You can eat hearty.

"For lunch, you can have mushrooms simmered with one teaspoon of marjoram and one of sage, or else sliced carrots and turnips boiled with a teaspoon of thyme and a bay leaf, or tomatoes fried in butter with a teaspoon of sage and a teaspoon of rosemary. That's your basic lunch, any one of those three. You get a second course, if you're not dieting to lose weight, of hard cheese or stewed pears with a teaspoonful of cinnamon, or rice pudding with lots and lots of allspice and ginger."

"Hey, those are healthy gobs of spice. A whole teaspoonful of each?"

"Well, that's where the sexiness comes from. Now, for dinner, you can have either a chicken roasted with a table-spoon of dried rosemary, plenty of parsley and lemon all rubbed inside the bird, or a steak fried with one teaspoonful of thyme ..." Seeing my smile he adds quickly, "That's *a vegetarian* steak of course. Your third choice is roast veal covered with one tablespoon of rosemary."

"But veal is meat, too."

"It's not red beef."

"No, but it's a baby beef."

"Well, if you're that rigid you can substitute fish rubbed with rosemary."

"Would you taste anything but the rosemary?"

"Don't knock it till you've tried it. You can have vegetables, too. Let's see, a small potato boiled in water with one-half a teaspoon of cumin seeds for each half-cup of water or boiled rice with half a teaspoon of marjoram, or cabbage boiled with half a teaspoon of cumin seed per cup of water."

"And for dessert?"

"You vary that, too. Apples or pears steamed with honey, lemon, and one teaspoon of cumin seed per apple, or a fresh fruit salad with lots of ginger—oh, yeah, and salads with the meal. Lettuce, and you make a dressing of lemon juice, olive oil, and a teaspoon of tarragon, or you can have a raw chopped vegetable salad with cumin seed."

"You're not pulling my leg? You really go on this diet? Seriously?" I ask him.

"I sure do. At least once a year, and sometimes even more often. What it does is clean out my system. I don't eat anything the first day, like I told you—just fruit juice and herbal tea. The second day, if I really want to lose weight, I have only some boiled rice and about half a cup of dry white wine. The third day I start the diet and stay on it—oh, about three days, maybe four, five. My body tells me when I've had enough. Everything in me wakes up. I come alive and I look at things differently. And sex—Man! That is far out. You can just feel the sexual strength in you."

"And the itching genital tract?"

Sheldon looks hurt. "I'm talking seriously and you make jokes. Look, you tell Frank and Amber to switch to my love diet. It may not take off as much weight as theirs, but on the other hand, it may give them so much exercise they'll *work* the weight off!"

> *Fresh herbs are best for this diet because of their rich flavor and aroma. Dried herbs can also be used, but remember to use less to make up for their more concentrated taste.*

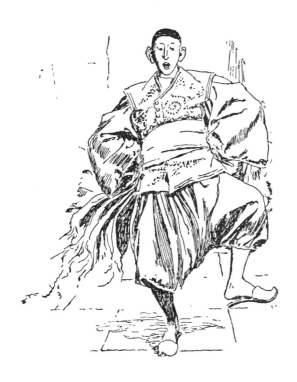

LAST CHANTS
FOR PEACE OF MIND

This ancient technique can help you clear your mind for the important things you want to think about.

A group of us were coming home from the theater one summer night when we passed a city corner where a band of yellow-robed mock Hindus with bald heads shuffled through a monotonous dance step chanting *Hare Krishna, Hare Krishna, Krishna, Krishna, Hare, Hare, Hare Rama, Hare Rama, Rama, Rama, Hare, Hare,* over and over as we stood there.

One of the group, a nonchanter with tennis sneakers under his saffron skirts, and a dark stubble on his gaunt, shaved head, came round with a cup to collect meager contributions.

Later, over coffee in a nearby café, Henry shook his head. "I wouldn't give them a cent. Freaks, the bunch of them!"

"I don't know," his wife Lila said thoughtfully. "There's something very soothing about that chant. Hare, Hare, Hare Rama—It keeps going round and round in my head."

"Like a whatchamacallit," Shelly said. "One of those mnemonics? Is that the name? Those things that keep you from thinking?"

Arthur, the professor in our group, lit a cigarette and said, "You've hit it there, Shelly. Wrong word, but chanting is a way to keep you from thinking. The words of the chant force out any logical thought. If the chant is constructed properly, it resonates through your head. The Krishna chant is a very effective one. It fills the resonance pockets in your skull and blocks out any thinking."

"But what's the sense of that?" I ask curiously. "Why block out thinking?"

"Meditation blocks out thinking. Transcendental meditation is a device to keep you from thinking. There the chant is reduced to one mantra you repeat over and over, but a good chant does the same thing. It pushes all thought aside and with it the bother of thought, the nagging anxiety of thinking."

"I've never heard thinking described like that." Henry laughed. "You make it sound as if thinking were something bad, something to avoid."

"Sometimes it is. Sometimes you want to clear your head of all the dusty cobwebs of thought. Chanting can do that, and it can also let you turn on, get high without drugs."

"Get high?" Lila asked doubtfully.

"It can give you a psychic high," Arthur insisted. "The repetition of sound and tone and a changed method of breathing increases the oxygen level of the blood to the brain. You alter your consciousness."

"Do you need the yellow robes and sneakers with sweat socks?" Henry asked distastefully. "Those kids just turn me off!"

"Of course you don't need all that," Arthur said. "With

them chanting's part of a religion, but you don't have to be religious to chant—or even have a mantra."

"What is a mantra?" Lila asked. "I keep hearing people use the term, and I honestly don't know what it means."

"It's any sort of sound. It's supposed to be the sound of the universe, and a good mantra stimulates or arouses a sympathetic vibration in the chest and head, but you can use any word as a mantra. Try *one* over and over. *One, one, one, one*—It gradually loses meaning as a word and begins vibrating in your head. Or take any name. I could use mine—*Arthur, Arthur, Arthur*—again it loses all meaning and becomes a vibrating sound."

"But a sound that reverberates is better for a mantra," I said thoughtfully. "I've heard of a Tantric yoga chant that goes *Live Very Richly You Happy One*."

"That doesn't sound to me as if it would reverberate," Shelly said, shaking her head."

"No, no—" I explained. "You don't chant that. There are six words in the title and each stands for an energy center along the spine. For each center you take the first letter of each word in the chant and add *un*. Un is very, you know, resonant. Start with the L for live and add it to un. That's *Lun*. Chant that for five minutes, then go on to *Vun, Run, Yun, Hun and Oun*. Chant each one for five minutes. The chanting is supposed to move the energy up your spine to your head as you go."

We sat around the table then, softly humming *Lun, Lun, Lun* ... When the waitress came to take our order we broke off in embarrassment, asked for coffee and danish, and watched her walk away unperturbed.

"Do you really think chanting is useful?" Lila asked.

"Well, that depends," Arthur said thoughtfully. "It depends on what use you put it to. It can be soothing and pleasing, and by driving all thought out it can bring the same calm meditation does. You know," he added after a pause, "what you were saying about the energy center in the spine reminds me of another type of chant called body chanting."

"What's that?"

"It's a spinal chant. It needs two people, a chanter and I

guess a chantee. The chantee lies on his stomach on the floor, his arms at his side while the chanter bends over him and puts his lips about an inch from the chantee's spine. He starts near the tailbone and chants for five minutes, one word, like your *Vun, Vun, Vun*—over and over, then he moves up to another spot for another five minutes. He covers six key spots in all and ends at the head."

Shelly shivered. "I get chills just thinking about it. What's supposed to happen?"

"I've had it done to me and it's really very sensational. I can't explain it, but there's a deep, vibratory quality, especially if the chanter has a deep bass voice. It causes some sort of trembling in your spine and it seems to release a flow of energy up your backbone. It's really extraordinary. You get up and feel completely recharged for hours."

Lila shook her head. "It sounds very intimate. I can't think of anyone but a husband or lover chanting up my backbone!"

"You know," Shelly said thoughtfully. "All this chanting is very close to praying."

"How do you mean?"

"I can go to church and kneel down, especially in a beautiful church with stained glass windows and big, open spaces—the churches where you get a sense of awe—and I feel that if I pray repetitively, saying the same prayer over and over, like a penance after confession, if I keep at it, especially in Latin where it becomes a mechanical formula, after a while it does just what Arthur says a chant does. It recharges me and gives me a peculiar high. I come out feeling tremendously refreshed. I've always put that feeling down to absolving my sins, the confession and the penance, but now I wonder if it could be the act of praying itself?"

"We have a similar thing in synagogue," Henry said thoughtfully. "Especially on the High Holy Days. I attend an Orthodox synagogue and we pray in Hebrew. I don't really understand the language, though I read it fluently . . ."

"What?" Arthur stubbed out his cigarette and stared at him. "You've got to explain that."

"It's very common among Jews. We learn to read Hebrew

phonetically. We read it to pray, and in synagogue we read
passage after passage without knowing what we're saying. At
least that's true of my generation. Nowadays they may teach it
as a language. But I tell you, a few hours of reading it for me,
and I get the exact same high that Shelly describes from
church—a cleansing, exhilarating feeling."

We sat silently, considering that while our coffee and
danish came, then, as we started to eat, Shelly said, "I'm really
surprised at you, Henry."

"Why?"

"For putting the Krishna boys down. They're really into the
same thing as we are—chanting to get a religious high!"

Considering that carefully, we all look out the coffee shop
windows to where the dim, yellow robes of the Krishna
dancers are still visible, leaping up and down in the dusk.